Sex Talk

The Ultimate Collection of Ribald, Raunchy, and Provocative Quotations

James Wolfe

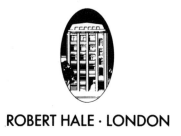

ROBERT HALE · LONDON

© *James Wolfe 1995*
First published in Great Britain 1995

Published by arrangement with Carol Publishing Group Inc.
600 Madison Avenue, New York, NY, USA

ISBN 0 7090 5708 3

Robert Hale Limited
Clerkenwell House
Clerkenwell Green
London EC1R 0HT

2 4 6 8 10 9 7 5 3 1

Printed in Great Britain by
St Edmundsbury Press Limited, Bury St Edmunds, Suffolk
and bound by WBC Book Manufacturers Limited

Contents

Introduction

L ibrary shelves are crammed with books of quotations. Many are compilations of quotes on a variety of subjects. Some are concerned with quotes by specific subsets of society such as various ethnic groups, women, or homosexuals. Others deal with specific topics like sports, politics, or business. There are obviously quote books which include sex and related topics, but there is no quote book that concentrates as exclusively and exhaustively as this book on the one subject we all find most interesting—sex.

Approximately 1,400 raunchy, controversial, thought-provoking, outrageous, humorous, and thoroughly entertaining statements by rock, movie, and sports celebrities, politicians and statesmen, generals, writers, philosophers, scientists, scholars, and other notables are contained in this volume. Over seven hundred different authors are included in the book, representing a tremendous diversity of background and perspective, from Plato to Presley, Eleanor to Hillary, Napoleon to Haig, Welk to Rose—Axl, that is. Celebrities are amazingly frank in discussing sexual matters, including such typically private information as sexual fantasies, preferences, and prowess; gossip about friends and foes; love in marriage and extramaritally. Gleeful, reflective, and regretful confessions concerning infidelity, orgasms, promiscuity, voyeurism, and virtue, as well as, advice to the lovelorn from ancient Greek philosophers, are all shamelessly included in this volume.

The collection of quotations is organized into 89 categories, alphabetized by author within each category. The categories range from advice to women's lib and include anatomy, battle of the sexes, erogenous zones, first times, family values, homosexuality, horniness, ideal partners, love and marriage, kinky and oral sex, seduction, and toys. The complete list of categories is outlined in the table of contents. An index provides easy access to each quotation author and includes a brief description of each author's career or claim to fame.

Quotations for this work were selected for a variety of reasons. The attempt was made to be objective in the selection process and not allow personal biases or political preferences to intrude into the selection of quotes. The views included in the book span all sides of the political spectrum—from the far right, such as Ronald Reagan, Pat Buchanan, and Rush Limbaugh, to as far left as Timothy Leary and Jane Fonda. Other biases were kept out of the selection equation as much as consciously possible. Although much thought went into the selection of each individual statement, the process still has to be described as qualitative. In other words, if it appealed to me, made me laugh or cringe, it is probably included. The following factors were considered in selecting items:

• Significance: Is the statement important or said by someone so important that the statement takes on significance?

• Provocative: Is it thought-provoking or controversial or does it represent a new way of viewing an old problem?

• Gossip or voyeuristic value: Is the statement sufficiently juicy or outrageous?

• Humor: If it made me laugh, it is in; if I smiled,

perhaps additional criteria for inclusion were considered as well.

• Entertaining: Is the quotation interesting or was it said by someone who is interesting; does it provide a historical perspective or say something about our society?

In summary, many of the quotes are highly significant, provocative, or humorous. Many are attributed to significant people; this was a major consideration for selection. But some are not. No claims are made with respect to social or educational value or any individual quote or the collection in total. The overriding criteria was entertainment value.

The quotes were collected from hundreds of sources. Books, magazines, interviews, radio, and television, and the work of other compilers were reviewed. Each quote is assumed to be accurate, and considerable effort was made to check each quote, but I cannot warrant the accuracy of all my sources. All quotations were obtained from previously published or broadcast sources. The quotes are, of course, the opinions of those who first spoke or wrote them.

Developing this book has been a pleasurable journey which I hope you will enjoy as much as I have.

Advice

Never eat at a place called Mom's. Never play cards with a man named Doc. And never lie down with a woman who's got more troubles than you have.

—Nelson Algren

Nine cases out of ten, a woman had better show more affection than she feels.

—Jane Austen

Try everything once except incest and folk dancing.

—Sir Thomas Beecham

Do it quick, my wife would say, get it over as fast as you can. It's not nice.

—The Boston Strangler

You can add years to your life by wearing your pants backwards.

—Johnny Carson

There are two guidelines in good sex: don't do anything you really don't enjoy, and find out your partner's needs and don't balk if you can help it.

—Alex Comfort

Take off the shell with your clothes.

—Alex Comfort

Be careful what you show—and what you don't show.
—Marlene Dietrich

Never go to bed mad. Stay up and fight.
—Phyllis Diller

You should never attempt to outwit a woman.
—Alexandre Dumas

Thou shalt not commit adultery.
—Exodus 20

Never try to impress a woman, because if you do she'll expect you to keep up to the standard for the rest of your life.
—W. C. Fields

He that displays too often his wife and his wallet is in danger of having both of them borrowed.
—Ben Franklin

There are three secrets my mother told me. Be a maid in the living room, a cook in the kitchen, and a whore in the bedroom. I figure so long as I have a maid and a cook, I'll do the rest myself.
—Jerry Hall

Never get married in the morning, because you may never know who you'll meet that night.
—Paul Hornung

When a woman is speaking to you, listen to what she says with her eyes.
—Victor Hugo

2

Just remember, as long as you don't hurt anybody, or talk badly about them, or take advantage of them sexually, you'll always be disappointedly dull.
                                    —Eric Idle

The only unnatural sex act is that which you cannot perform,
                                    —Alfred Kinsey

Sleep around all you want but don't get married.
                                    —Debra Koenig advising
                                      seventh grade girls on Take
                                      Your Daughter to Work Day

All married couples should learn the art of battle as they should learn the art of making love.
                                    —Ann Landers

If you want to improve sex, ask, "What do you enjoy? What do you feel? Because I care."
                                    —William Masters

You must not force sex to do the work of love or love to do the work of sex.
                                    —Mary McCarthy

Candy is dandy, but liquor is quicker.
                                    —Ogden Nash

If the wife comes through as being too strong and too intelligent, it makes the husband look like a wimp.
                                    —Richard M. Nixon advising Bill
                                      Clinton in the 1992 campaign

Women, let the pleasure penetrate even to the marrow of your bones, and let the enjoyment be equally divided between you and your lover. Whisper tender words, murmur softly and licentious suggestions to sharpen your sweet sport.
>—Ovid

If your posterior is cute, let it be seen from behind.
>—Ovid

When you have found the place where a woman loves to be fondled, don't you be ashamed to touch it any more than she is.
>—Ovid

Women can always be caught; that's the first rule of the game.
>—Ovid

Do not let too strong a light come into your bedroom. There are in a beauty a great many things which are enhanced by being seen only in a half-light.
>—Ovid

Go very lightly on the vices, such as carrying on in society. The social ramble ain't restful.
>—Satchell Paige on staying young

Trust your husband, adore your husband, and get as much as you can in your own name.
>—Advice to Joan Rivers from her mother

There are two rules to living well. The first is, don't sweat the little shit. The second is, it's all little shit.
—David Lee Roth

Never trust a husband too far or a bachelor too near.
—Helen Rowland

You must lay down the treasures of your body.
—William Shakespeare in
Measure for Measure

Don't play no faggots.
—Sylvester Stallone advising a
fellow actor

Copulation is dangerous immediately after a meal and during the two or three hours which the first digestion needs, or having finished a rapid walk or any other violent exercise. In the same way, if the mental faculties are excited by some mental effort, by a theater party or dance, rest is necessary, and it is advisable to defer amatory experience till the next morning.
—Physician Bernard Talmey
advising in 1919

Wear it anywhere you want to be touched.
—Elizabeth Taylor on a new
cologne for men

Regard the society of women as a necessary unpleasantness of social life, and avoid it as much as possible.
—Leo Tolstoy

Never kick a fresh turd on a hot day.
—Harry S. Truman

My advice to girls: first, don't smoke—to excess; second, don't drink—to excess; third, don't marry—to excess.
—Mark Twain

Accept every blind date you can get, even with a girl who wears jeans. Maybe you can talk her out of them.
—Abigail Van Buren

Don't stint on the foreplay. Be inventive.
—Dr. Ruth Westheimer

Satisfy your partner even when you may not feel like sex.
—Dr. Ruth Westheimer

Nothing risqué, nothing gained.
—Alexander Woollcott

Aging

The only thing I regret about my life is the length of it. If I had to live my life again, I'd make all the same mistakes—only sooner.
—Tallulah Bankhead

Sex after ninety is like trying to shoot pool with a rope. Even putting my cigar in its holder is a thrill.
—George Burns

I'd go out with women my age, but there are no women my age.

—George Burns

I have my eighty-seventh birthday coming up and people ask me what I'd most appreciate getting. I'll tell you: a paternity suit.

—George Burns

Getting married and getting old are the two things that save everybody's ass.

—Cher

An archaeologist is the best husband a woman can have. The older she gets, the more interested he is in her.

—Agatha Christie

I'm at the age where food has taken the place of sex in my life. In fact, I've just had a mirror put over my kitchen table.

—Rodney Dangerfield

As a young man I used to have four supple members and a stiff one. Now I have four stiff and a supple one.

—Henri duc d'Aumale

Older women are best because they always think they may be doing it for the last time.

—Ian Fleming

As they get on, after five or six years, in most married couples, the old feeling begins to dissipate. Food oftentimes takes the place of sex in a relationship.

—Alfred Hitchcock

I've been around so long I can remember Doris Day before she was a virgin.

—Groucho Marx

I don't miss sex. I know I can't do it properly anymore.

—Groucho Marx

A man is only as old as the woman he feels.

—Groucho Marx

I think in twenty years I'll be looked at like Bob Hope. Doing these President jokes and golf shit. It scares me.

—Eddie Murphy

First you forget names, then you forget faces; then you forget to zip your fly, then you forget to unzip your fly.

—Branch Rickey

I don't want to be horny when I'm seventy, because it will be so hard to fulfill.

—Neil Simon

Women may be the only group that grows more radical with age.

—Gloria Steinem

From birth to eighteen, a girl needs good parents; from eighteen to thirty-five she needs good looks; from thirty-five to fifty-five she needs a good personality; and from fifty-five on she needs cash.

—Sophie Tucker

For certain people, after fifty, litigation takes the place of sex.

—Gore Vidal

At seventy, I find orgasmic sex quite dispensable.
—Tennessee Williams

Now that I'm over sixty, I'm veering toward respectability.
—Shelley Winters

Americana

In America sex is an obsession, in other parts of the world it is a fact.
—Marlene Dietrich

The thing that impresses me the most about America is the way parents obey their children.
—The Duke of Windsor

Playboy is sex, closely linked to great business success— and those are the two great Puritan hang-ups.
—Hugh Hefner

The great American formula for sex is: a kiss on the lips, a hand on the breast, and a dive for the groin.
—William Masters

American women expect to find in their husbands the perfection that English women only hope to find in their butlers.
—W. Somerset Maugham

This country is into tits and ass.
—Neil Simon

Americans make love worse than any other race on earth.
—Walt Whitman

When I first saw the [Niagara] falls I was disappointed in the outline. Every American bride is taken there, and the sight must be one of the earliest, if not the keenest, disappointments of American married life.

—Oscar Wilde

Anatomy, Female

I used to be so top-heavy that I leaned forward.

—Loni Anderson

Everybody knows I've got bigger boobs than Carol Burnett.

—Julie Andrews

The legs aren't so beautiful. I just know what to do with them.

—Marlene Dietrich

The only parts left of my original body are my elbows.

—Phyllis Diller

There is no female mind. The brain is not an organ of sex. [You may] as well speak of a female liver.

—Charlotte Perkins Gilman

There are two reasons why I'm in show business, and I'm standing on both of them.

—Betty Grable

To read the newspapers and magazines, you would think we were almost worshiping the female bosom.

—Billy Graham

The worst name anyone can be called is cunt. The best thing a cunt can be is small and unobtrusive: the anxiety about the bigness of the penis is only equaled by the anxiety about the smallness of the cunt. No woman wants a twat like a horsecollar.

—Germaine Greer

There are two good reasons why men will go to see her.

—Howard Hughes on actress
Jane Russell

I have everything I had twenty years ago, only it's a little lower.

—Gypsy Rose Lee

If God wanted us to think with our wombs, why did He give us brains?

—Claire Booth Luce

Really that little deelybob is too far away from the hole. It should be built right in.

—Loretta Lynn on the female
sex organ

Anyone who says he can see through women is missing a lot.

—Groucho Marx

The evidence indicates that woman is, on the whole, biologically superior to man.

—Ashley Montagu

[The adman] has discovered the vagina and it's like the next thing going. What happened is that the adman ran out of parts of the body. So the adman sat back and said, "What's left?" And some smart guy said, "The vagina!"
—David Ogilvy

And here they are, Jayne Mansfield.
—Jack Parr introducing Ms. Mansfield

I do have big tits. Always had them—pushed them up, whacked them around. Why not make fun of them? I've made a fortune with them.
—Dolly Parton

Can you imagine anybody wanting to look this way for real?
—Dolly Parton

All you talk about is vaginas, vaginas, vaginas. I'm getting out of here.
—Jeanette Rankin to Margaret Sanger at a birth control meeting

God bless Fergie for bringing back boobs and hips. Every fat farm girl should kiss Sarah Ferguson's chubby thighs.
—Joan Rivers

Husbands think we should know where everything is— like the uterus is a tracking device. He asks me, "Roseanne, do we have any Chee-tos left?" Like he can't go over to the sofa cushion and lift it himself.
—Roseanne

I have a brain and a uterus, and I use both.
—Pat Schroeder

I can't stand to touch those plastic breasts.
—Donald Trump on ex-wife
Ivana's cosmetic surgery

It's not what you'd call a figure, is it?
—Twiggy on herself

Anatomy, General

I'd rather see a man with his breast showing than a woman.
—Muhammad Ali

Sex is a pleasurable exercise in plumbing, but be careful or you'll get yeast in your drainpipe.
—Rita Mae Brown

The genitals themselves have not undergone the development of the rest of the human form in the direction of beauty.
—Sigmund Freud

Whoever named it necking was a poor judge of anatomy.
—Groucho Marx

It must be admitted that we English have sex on the brain, which is a very unfortunate place to have it.
—Malcolm Muggeridge

As I look around the West End these days, it seems that outside every thin girl is a fat man, trying to get in.
—Katherine Whitehorn

Anatomy, Male

My brain is my second favorite organ.
—Woody Allen

Erection is chiefly caused by scuraum, eringos, cresses, crymon, parsnips, artichokes, turnips, asparagus, candied ginger, acorns bruised to powder and drunk in muscatel, scallion, sea shellfish, etc.
—Aristotle

A man is two people, himself and his cock. A man always takes his friend to the party. Of the two, the friend is the nicer, being more able to show his feelings.
—Beryl Bainbridge

An erection at will is the moral equivalent of a valid credit card.
—Alex Comfort

Some men say their erections aren't as big as they recall them once being. But then their partner says, "Well, dear, you overestimated them back then too."
—Dr. Paul T. Costa Jr. on male menopause

The penis confers with human intelligence and has intelligence itself...and takes its own course...without license of thought by man.
—Leonardo da Vinci

14

Man is in the wrong in being ashamed to exhibit it...when he ought to adorn and display it.
—Leonardo da Vinci

The penis is the only muscle a man has that he cannot flex. It is also the only extremity that he cannot control....But even worse as it affects the dignity of its owner, in its seeming obedience to that inferior thing, woman. It rises at the sight, or even the thought of a woman.
—Elizabeth Gould Davis

Don't forget, the penis is mightier than the sword.
—Jay Hawkins

I still have a diary entry asking myself whether talk about the size of the male organ isn't a homosexual preoccupation: if things aren't too bad in other ways, I doubt any woman cares very much.
—Lillian Hellman

It's almost impossible to judge the size of an erect penis from its appearance in the flaccid state.
—Xaviera Hollander

Beware of the man who denounces women writers; his penis is tiny and cannot spell.
—Erica Jong

A stiff cock is nothing to be ashamed of.
—Linda Lovelace

I'm going to Iowa for an award, Carnegie Hall, to France to be honored. I'd give it all up for one erection.
—Groucho Marx

I just wanted to see what it looked like in the spotlight.
—Jim Morrison on why he
exposed himself on stage

When the Dow-Jones Average goes up, the penis will too.
—John O'Connor

I wonder why men get serious at all. They have this delicate long thing hanging outside their bodies which goes up and down by its own will. If I were a man I would always be laughing at myself.
—Yoko Ono

Bathroom

Neil Armstrong was the first man to walk on the moon. I am the first man to piss his pants on the moon.
—Buzz Aldren

My wife is an immature woman. I would be home in the bathroom taking a bath and my wife would walk in whenever she felt like it and sink my boats.
—Woody Allen

I have come to the conclusion that a good set of bowels is worth more to a man than any quantity of brains.
—Josh Billings

A man can go seventy years without a piece of ass, but he can die in a week without a bowel movement.
—Charles Bukowski

The toilets. They're real nice.

—Darren Daulton on what he
likes best about Baltimore's
new baseball stadium

If the husband and wife can possibly afford it, they should definitely have separate bathrooms for the sake of the marriage.

—Doris Day

The trouble with being a princess is that it is so hard to have a pee.

—Princess Diana

Lobbing one into the men's room at the Kremlin.

—Barry Goldwater in the 1964
presidential campaign about
the use of nuclear weapons

We have all passed a lot of water since then.

—Sam Goldwyn

In a way, I'm glad to know the place I used to shit will be Henry's office.

—Bryce N. Harlow, Nixon aid,
on giving up his bathroom to
expand Henry Kissinger's
office

I grew up with six brothers. That's how I learned to dance—waiting to get into the bathroom.

—Bob Hope

I'm a loner. I like a good meal, a good script, and a good BM. That to me is a great life.

—Jack Klugman

Sitting on the toilet peeing—that's where I have my most contemplative moments.

—Madonna

I don't like to be bugged in bathrooms. I mean, people hand me cassettes under the stall. It's brutal.

—Bonnie Raitt

Battle of the Sexes

I married beneath me. All women do.

—Lady Nancy Astor

The way to fight a woman is with your hat—grab it and run.

—John Barrymore

When archaeologists discover the missing arms of Venus de Milo, they will find she was wearing boxing gloves.

—John Barrymore

Woman would be more charming if one could fall into her arms without falling into her hands.

—Ambrose Bierce

Women have two weapons—cosmetics and tears.

—Napoleon Bonaparte

Girls have an unfair advantage over men; if they can't get what they want by being smart, they can get it by being dumb.

—Yul Brynner

There will always be a battle between the sexes because men and women want different things. Men want women and women want men.

—George Burns

Men don't like independent women.

—Shirley Chisholm

My message to men is, "Don't screw around with women because they can turn around and screw you back."

—Jackie Collins

Being a woman is a terribly difficult trade, since it consists principally of dealing with men.

—Joseph Conrad

Most women set out to change a man, and when they have changed him they do not like him.

—Marlene Dietrich

Woman inspires us to great things and prevents us from achieving them.

—Alexandre Dumas

You see an awful lot of smart guys with dumb women, but hardly ever see a smart woman with a dumb guy.

—Clint Eastwood

God made men stronger but not necessarily more intelligent. He gave women intuition and femininity. And, used properly, that combination easily jumbles the brain of any man I've ever met.

—Farrah Fawcett

Man has his will—but woman has her way.
—Oliver Wendell Holmes

Men and women, women and men. It will never work.
—Erica Jong

Women are the only exploited group in history to have been idealized into powerlessness.
—Erica Jong

If anyone is exploited by *Penthouse*, it's men. Women are paid handsomely to appear in the magazine, while men have to pay for the privilege of seeing them.
—Kathy Keeton

Nobody will ever win the battle of the sexes. There's too much fraternizing with the enemy.
—Henry Kissinger

Women who seek to be equal to men lack ambition.
—Timothy Leary

All men laugh at the Three Stooges and all women think that the Three Stooges are assholes.
—Jay Leno

The only way to resolve a situation with a girl is to jump on her.
—Lee Marvin

Women want mediocre men and men are working to be as mediocre as possible.
—Margaret Mead

Men have a much better time of it than women; for one thing, they marry later; for another, they die earlier.
—H. L. Mencken

On one issue at least, men and women agree; they both distrust women.
—H.L. Mencken

Given half a chance, a woman offers her whole being. It's instinctive with her. Not a man! A man is always more muddled than a woman. He needs a woman for no other purpose than to be straightened out. Sometimes it takes nothing more than a good, clean, healthy fuck to do the trick.
—Henry Miller

The cleverest woman on earth is the biggest fool on earth with a man.
—Dorothy Parker

Men have taken my self-esteem and flushed it away; it's somewhere in the mid-Atlantic right now.
—Joan Rivers

It takes a woman twenty years to make a man of her son, and another woman twenty minutes to make a fool of him.
—Helen Rowland

My boyfriend and I broke up. He wanted to get married, and I didn't want him to.
—Rita Rudner

When men and women agree, it is only in their conclusions; their reasons are always different.
—George Santayana

Home is the girl's prison and the woman's workhouse.
—George Bernard Shaw

Once made equal to man, woman becomes his superior.
—Socrates

Why does a woman work ten years to change a man's habits and then complain that he's not the man she married?

—Barbra Streisand

A woman's place is in the wrong.
—James Thurber

The first time you buy a house you see how pretty the paint is and buy it. The second time you look to see if the basement has termites. It's the same with men.
—Lupe Velez

Men have been trained and conditioned by women, not unlike the way Pavlov conditioned his dogs, into becoming his slaves. As compensation for their labor, men are given the periodic use of women's vaginas.
—Esther Vilar

There aren't any hard women, just soft men.
—Raquel Welch

Whatever women do, they must do twice as well as men. Luckily, this is not difficult.
—Charlotte Whitton

Between men and women there is no friendship possible. There is passion, enmity, worship, love, but no friendship.
—Oscar Wilde

The only time a woman really succeeds in changing a man is when he's a baby.

—Natalie Wood

Beauty/Glamour

There are no really ugly women. Every woman is a Venus in her own way.

—Brigitte Bardot

...has a double chin and an overdeveloped chest and she's rather short in the leg. So I can hardly describe her as the most beautiful creature I've ever seen.

—Richard Burton on Elizabeth Taylor

The truth is, no ugly woman can succeed in politics.

—Edith Cresson

My breasts are beautiful, and I've got to tell you, they've gotten a lot of attention for what is relatively short screen time.

—Jamie Lee Curtis

All the doors automatically open for a beautiful woman. I know it's very fashionable for good-looking ladies to say how hard it is to be beautiful, but that's not true.

—Catherine Deneuve

When I go to the beauty parlor, I always use the emergency entrance. Sometimes I just go for an estimate.

—Phyllis Diller

Is it too much to ask that women be spared the daily struggle for superhuman beauty in order to offer it to the caresses of a subhumanly ugly mate?

—Germaine Greer

I rat the tar out jof it, spray the hell out of it. I get it up there and defy gravity.

—Gail Haitt, hairdresser for
Ann Richards, governor of
Texas

It's the plain women who know about love; the beautiful women are too busy being fascinating.

—Katharine Hepburn

All women think they're ugly, even pretty women. A man who understood this could fuck more women than Don Giovanni. They all think their cunts are ugly... they all find fault with their figures.

—Erica Jong

I'm tired of all this nonsense about beauty being only skin deep. That's deep enough. What do you want—an adorable pancreas?

—Jean Kerr

Any girl can be glamorous. All you have to do is stand still and look stupid.

—Hedy Lamarr

The best way to apply fragrance...is to spray it into the air...and walk into it.

—Estée Lauder

Glamour is where a man knows a woman is a woman.
—Gina Lollobrigida

No one ever called me pretty when I was a little girl.
—Marilyn Monroe

There is no such thing as an altogether ugly woman—or altogether beautiful.
—Michel Eyquem de Montaigne

There are no ugly women, only lazy ones.
—Helena Rubenstein

Birth

I have an intense desire to return to the womb. Anybody's.
—Woody Allen

Giving birth is like trying to push a piano through a transom.
—Alice Roosevelt Longworth

Perhaps a cunt, smelly though it may be, is one of the prime symbols for the connection between all things. To enter the world by way of the vagina is as good a way as any.
—Henry Miller

To my embarrassment, I was born in bed with a lady.
—Wilson Mizner

When I was giving birth the nurse asked, "Still think blonds have more fun?"

—Joan Rivers

Birth Control

Last night I discovered a new form of oral contraception—she said no.

—Woody Allen

We're more effective than birth control pills.

—Johnny Carson on late night
talk show hosts

When I was in the service, you didn't need birth control devices because all the WACs looked like William Bendix.

—Johnny Carson

It makes it possible for the sexual women to act like a sexual man.

—Dr. Marcus Crahan on the pill

Whenever I hear people discussing birth control, I always remember that I was the fifth.

—Clarence Darrow

It is now quite lawful for a Catholic woman to avoid pregnancy by resorting to mathematics, though she is still forbidden to resort to physics or chemistry.

—H. L. Mencken

My father really should have worn a condom. He did not deserve Howard Spira as a son.

—Howard Spira, who was
convicted of extorting from
George Steinbrenner

Women who miscalculate are called "mothers."

—Abigail Van Buren

Bisexuality

Bisexuality doubles your chances for a date on Saturday night.

—Woody Allen

A Bay Area bisexual told me I didn't quite coincide with either of his desires.

—Woody Allen

One of the nicest whatever you want to call it—loves of my life—was a woman. Being bisexual, you're very much looked down upon by the uppity members of gay lib.

—Joan Baez

If you swing both ways, you really swing...double your pleasure.

—Joan Baez

I had a lot of sex from the girls and queers around the neighborhood. Some of them was amazed at how I could come and then five minutes later come again. The queers loved that and would pay for it too. But it really was women, not any special one. Just women.

—The Boston Strangler

Like many men, I too have had homosexual experiences and I am not ashamed.

—Marlon Brando

Once you know what women are like, men get kind of boring. I'm not trying to put them down, I mean I like them sometimes as people, but sexually they're dull.

—Rita Mae Brown

I don't believe anyone is heterosexual. That idea is a load of crap. I've slept with girls and I've slept with boys.

—Boy George

OK, I've experimented with both sexes, but I'm not a limp-wristed floozy and I'm not a transvestite. I'm a very masculine person.

—Boy George

That was a part of the swinging period of the seventies—I was exploring the outer limits of my sexuality, and it included bisexuality. But I never really had an emotional connection with a man.

—Hugh Hefner

OK, OK. If you're asking me am I one, I'll go that route— good public relations. If it's good enough for Gore Vidal and Elton John, it's good enough for me. I am bisexual, happy and proud. A woman in every bed...and a man too.

—Rock Hudson

There's nothing wrong with going to bed with somebody of your own sex. People should be very free with sex—they should draw the line at goats.

—Elton John

Ever since I had that interview in which I said I was bisexual it seems twice as many people wave at me in the streets.

—Elton John

I haven't met anyone that I would like to settle down with—of either sex.

—Elton John

All of my sexual experiences when I was young were with girls. I mean we didn't have those sleep-overs for nothing. I think that's really normal; same-sex experimentation.

—Madonna

The time has come, I think, when we must recognize bisexuality as a normal form of human behavior.

—Margaret Mead

I got a girl in every port and a couple of guys in every port too.

—Sal Mineo

As far as I'm concerned, being any gender is a drag.

—Patti Smith

I was too polite to ask.

—Gore Vidal on whether his
first sex experience was
straight or gay

29

Censorship

If there is a bedrock principle underlying the First Amendment, it is that the government may not prohibit the expression of an idea simply because society finds the idea itself offensive or disagreeable.

—William J. Brennan Jr.

What's wrong with appealing to prurient interest? I really want the Supreme Court to tell me that fucking is dirty and no good.

—Lenny Bruce

Censorship is about stopping people reading or seeing what we do not want to read or see ourselves.

—Lord Diplock

We have a right to be tasteless under the First Amendment.

—Larry Flynt

Murder is a crime. Writing about it isn't. Sex is not a crime, but writing about it is. Why?

—Larry Flynt

I think movies have to be censored. Otherwise your child's mind will be corrupted.

—Jayne Mansfield

If the First Amendment means anything, it means that a state has no business telling a man, sitting alone in his own house, what books he may read or what films he may watch. Our whole constitutional heritage rebels at the thought of giving government the power to control men's minds.

—Thurgood Marshall

Scenes of passion...should not be introduced when not essential to the plot....In general, passion should be so treated that these scenes do not stimulate the lower and baser elements.

—Motion Picture Producers and
Distributors of America code
of March 31, 1930

Do not do unto others as you would that they should do unto you. Their tastes may not be the same as yours.

—George Bernard Shaw

Censorship reflects society's lack of confidence in itself.

—Potter Stewart

If a man is pictured chopping off a woman's breast, it only gets an "R" rating; but if, God forbid, a man is pictured kissing a woman's breast, it gets an "X" rating. Why is violence more acceptable than tenderness?

—Sally Struthers

I believe in censorship. After all, I made a fortune out of it.

—Mae West

Chastity/Virginity

Give me chastity, but not yet.
—Saint Augustine

Girls are always presuming I've kept my heterosexual virginity.
—David Bowie

Sometimes when I look at my children, I say to myself...you should have stayed a virgin.
—Lillian Carter

Filth and old age, I'm sure you agree, are powerful wardens upon chastity.
—Geoffrey Chaucer

We may eventually come to realize that chastity is no more a virtue than malnutrition.
—Alex Comfort

For me it will be enough that a marble stone should declare that a queen, having reigned such a time, lived and died a virgin.
—Queen Elizabeth I

A woman's chastity consists, like an onion, of a series of coats.
—Nathaniel Hawthorne

A chaste woman who teases is worse than a streetwalker.
—James G. Huneker

Chastity—the most unnatural of sexual perversions.
—Aldous Huxley

I'm still a nice Jewish girl who believes in saving it for the wedding night.
—Ann Landers

Nature abhors a virgin—a frozen asset.
—Claire Booth Luce

Losing my virginity was a career move.
—Madonna

How has it happened, what have we come to that the scarlet letter these days isn't *A*, but *V*?
—Joyce Maynard on virginity

Aren't women prudes if they don't and prostitutes if they do?
—Kate Millett

I think Gandhi is absolutely wrong...his advice can only lead to frustration, inhibition, neurosis, and all manner of physical and nervous ills.
—Jawaharlal Nehru on
Gandhi's advice on celibacy

Those who choose matrimony do well; those who choose virginity or voluntary abstinence do better.
—Pope John Paul II

I was married a virgin.

—Elizabeth Taylor

Clothes

They can have my falsies, pasties, and body stockings anytime.

—Candice Bergen

It's a historic moment for our company and for athletic supporters in general.

—Randy Black on Bike Athletic
Company's 300 millionth
jockstrap

You can't get snot off a suede jacket.

—Lenny Bruce

In my day hot pants were something we had, not wore.

—Bette Davis

I dress for women and undress for men.

—Angie Dickinson

Contrary to popular belief, English women do not wear tweed nightgowns.

—Hermione Gingold

Your dresses should be tight enough to show you're a woman and loose enough to show you're a lady.

—Edith Head

Seamed stockings aren't subtle but they certainly do the job. You shouldn't wear them when out with someone you're not prepared to sleep with, since their presence is tantamount to saying, "Hi there, big fellow, please rip my clothes off at your earliest opportunity." If you really want your escort paralytic with lust, stop frequently to adjust the seams.

—Cynthia Heimel

It is difficult to see why lace should be so expensive; it's mostly holes.

—Mary Wilson Little

A beautiful woman seductively dressed will never catch cold no matter how low cut her gown.

—Friedrich Nietzsche

Sex is a bad thing because it rumples the clothes.

—Jackie Kennedy Onassis

Brevity is the soul of lingerie.

—Dorothy Parker

It's a good thing I was born a female, or I'd have been a drag queen.

—Dolly Parton

I base most of my fashion taste on what doesn't itch.

—Gilda Radner

I haven't the figure for jeans.

—Margaret Thatcher

Clothes make the man. Naked people have little or no influence on society.

—Mark Twain

I tend to wear outfits that match the walls.

—Debra Winger

Plunging necklines attract more attention and cost less money.

—Shelley Winters

Cohabitation

You don't really know a person until you live with him, not just sleep with him. I staunchly believe no two people should get married until they have lived together. The young people have it right.

—Doris Day

Sometimes I wonder if men and women really suit each other. Perhaps they should live next door and just visit now and then.

—Katharine Hepburn

If married couples did not live together, happy marriages would be more frequent.

—Friedrich Nietzche

Confessions

I consider myself the zenith of sexual perversion.

—Woody Allen

36

Sometimes I'm so sweet even I can't stand it.
—Julie Andrews

I'm as pure as the driven slush.
—Tallulah Bankhead

I really am a cat transformed into a woman...I purr. I scratch. And sometimes I bite.
—Brigitte Bardot

It's impossible to be more flat chested than I am.
—Candice Bergen

I never loved a man I liked, and never liked a man I loved.
—Fanny Brice

The most romantic thing any woman ever said to me in bed was, "Are you sure you're not a cop?"
—Larry Brown

Sex, like baseball and dancing, was an area I was not likely to shine.
—Dick Cavett

Sometimes I feel like an old hooker.
—Cher

I do not look upon myself as a great lover. I just want to make people happy. Mind you, the fellow who can make a pretty girl laugh.
—Maurice Chevalier

To me inspiration and creativity come only when I have abstained from a woman for a longish period. When, with passion, I have emptied my fluid into a woman until I am pumped dry, then inspiration shuns me....The same forces which go to fertilize a woman and create a human being go to create a work of art.

—Frederic Chopin

When I prepare to go to sleep, everything comes off or out.

—Phyllis Diller

I never sleep with anyone. I never sleep when I have sex.

—Boy George

If a guy comes up to me and says "I know you," the first thing I think is, "Did he and I make it once?"

—Lee Grant

I am very upset and ashamed.

—Tonya Harding, explaining photos of her wearing a topless bridal gown.

I feel like a kid in the world's biggest candy store.

—Hugh Hefner

At one time I was considered quite sexless.

—Katharine Hepburn

I have been going braless for years. This delights my lover, although my mother still disapproves.

—Xaviera Hollander

Acting is not very hard. The most important things are being able to laugh and cry. If I have to cry, I think about my sex life. And if I have to laugh, well, I think of my sex life.

—Glenda Jackson on her acting technique

I can't get to sleep unless I've had a lay.
—John F. Kennedy

I love men, I love sex, and I don't care who knows it.
—Margot Kidder

I have one vice...it is not to be able to say no. Thank God for not making me a woman, but if He had, I suppose He would have made me just as ugly as He did, and no one would ever have tempted me.
—Abraham Lincoln

I've never owned a vibrator.
—Madonna

I've made an ass of myself so many times I often wonder if I am one.
—Norman Mailer

Let's just say I've gotten laughs in bed.
—Steve Martin

With all my white dresses, it wouldn't look nice to be dark down there. You could see through...It burns and sometimes I get these infections. But what else can I do?
—Marilyn Monroe on bleaching her pubic hair

My ass is way too big.
—Marilyn Monroe

I started as a dumb blond whore. I'll end as one.
—Marilyn Monroe

I'm buzzed by the female mystique.
—Jack Nicholson

Three minutes of serious fucking and I need eight hours of sleep and a bowl of Wheaties.
—Richard Pryor

In private life, I'm just a shallow, calculating bitch looking for a rich Arab to take me away.
—Joan Rivers

After we made love he took a piece of chalk and made an outline of my body.
—Joan Rivers

I left high school a virgin.
—Tom Selleck

I was too shy to express my sexual needs except over the phone to someone I don't know.
—Gary Shandling

I understand women perhaps because I have a very effeminate streak.
—Rod Stewart

I don't pretend to be an ordinary housewife.
—Elizabeth Taylor

The brute fact is that I am not and never have been a passionate lover....I want a healthy woman to steady my nerves and leave my mind free for real things.

—H. G. Wells

I used to be Snow White, but I drifted.

—Mae West

Almost from day one, my feelings toward Florence were more carnal than maternal.

—Barry Williams on his stage mom Florence Henderson in the TV show *The Brady Bunch*

I'm the modern, intelligent, independent-type woman. In other words, a girl who can't get a man.

—Shelley Winters

Crime/Violence

Outside of the killings, we have one of the lowest crime rates in the country.

—Marion Barry, mayor of Washington, D.C.

This is virgin territory for whorehouses.

—Al Capone on suburbia

When you have them by the balls, their hearts and minds will soon follow.

—Sign posted in Charles Colson's office

What he does on his own time is up to him.

—Harlon Copeland, county
sheriff, on a deputy caught
exposing himself in public

I'd like to thank my family for loving me and taking care of me. And the rest of the world can kiss my ass.

—Last words of Johnny Frank
Garrett before being
executed

You just give me the word and I'll turn that fucking island into a parking lot.

—Alexander Haig advising
Ronald Reagan on Cuba

I acted to show my love for Jody Foster.

—John Hinckley Jr. on why he
shot Ronald Reagan

He's come to realize this was an inappropriate way to impress a girl.

—Frederick Schwartz on John
Hinckley, Jr.

A life is more valuable than a penis.

—Lisa Kemler, defense attorney
for Lorena Bobbitt

A life such as John Bobbitt's is more valuable with a penis.

—Rush Limbaugh

How about cow dung at five paces.

—Abraham Lincoln when told to
choose his weapon for a duel

Sex is not only a divine and beautiful activity: it's a murderous activity. People kill each other in bed. Some of the greatest crimes ever committed were committed in bed. And no weapons were used.

—Norman Mailer

If the sex laws were applied drastically, I wonder who the jailers would be.

—William Masters

[Adult erotica] does not bear a relationship to rape and other acts of sexual violence.

—The Meese Commission

I don't give a shit what happens. I want you all to stonewall it, let them plead the Fifth Amendment, cover up or anything else, if it will save it, save the plan.

—Richard M. Nixon on the
Watergate cover-up

How much fame, money, and power does a woman have to achieve on her own before you can punch her in the face?

—P. J. O'Rourke

I just love a good fight. I'd rather fight than make love.

—Mr. T

It's only horny people who shoot people. I mean, you never feel aggressive just after you've gotten laid.

—Ted Turner

Women—you can't live with them, you can't shoot them.
—Steven Wright

Death

I believe in sex and death—two experiences that come once in a lifetime.
—Woody Allen

The difference between sex and death is death you do alone and no one is going to make fun of you.
—Woody Allen

The late porn star Johnny Holmes claimed to have been laid 14,000 times. He died of friction.
—Larry Brown

Sex isn't necessary. You won't die without it, but you can die with it.
—W. C. Fields

There are two days when a woman is a pleasure: the day one marries her and the day one buries her.
—Hipponax

Your food stamps will be stopped effective March 1992 because we received notice that you have passed away. May God bless you. You may reapply if there is a change in your circumstances.
—Letter from a social services office to a dead South Carolina man

Goddammit! He beat me to it.
> —Janis Joplin on Jimi Hendrix's death

There will be sex after death, we just won't be able to feel it.
> —Lily Tomlin

Divorce

For a while we pondered whether to take a vacation or get a divorce. We decided that a trip to Bermuda is over in two weeks, but a divorce is something you always have.
> —Woody Allen

The night before, Burt told me I was the love of his life...The next morning I was served with divorce papers.
> —Loni Anderson

The difference between divorce and legal separation is that legal separation gives a husband time to hide his money.
> —Johnny Carson

I'm a marvelous housekeeper. Every time I leave a man, I keep his house.
> —Zsa Zsa Gabor

Getting divorced just because you don't love a man is almost as silly as getting married just because you do.
> —Zsa Zsa Gabor

You never really know a man until you have divorced him.
> —Zsa Zsa Gabor

Conrad Hilton was very generous to me in the divorce settlement. He gave me 5,000 Gideon Bibles.
—Zsa Zsa Gabor

I don't think I'll get married again. I'll just find a woman I don't like and give her a house.
—Lewis Grizzard

I couldn't see tying myself down to a middle-aged woman with four children, even though the woman was my wife and the children were my own.
—Joseph Heller

There are four stages to a marriage. First there's the affair, then marriage, then children, and finally the fourth stage, without which you cannot know a woman, the divorce.
—Norman Mailer

She cried, and the judge wiped her tears on my checkbook.
—Tommy Manville

I'm getting a divorce and dating a much younger woman. There's no way I can keep my wife and my girlfriend happy at the same time.
—Ted Turner

If men acted after marriage as they do during courtship, there would be fewer divorces—and more bankruptcies.
—Frances Rodman

Always get married early in the morning. That way if it doesn't work out, you haven't wasted a whole day.
—Mickey Rooney

When I meet a man I ask myself, "Is this the man I want my children to spend the weekends with?"
—Rita Rudner

My divorce came as a complete surprise to me. That will happen when you haven't been home in eighteen years.
—Lee Trevino

Why do Jewish divorces cost so much? Because they are worth it.
—Henny Youngman

Drugs

Beer is not a good cocktail party drink, especially in a home where you don't know where the bathroom is.
—Billy Carter

I didn't inhale.
—Bill Clinton

'Twas a woman who drove me to drink, and I never had the courtesy to thank her for it.
—W. C. Fields

Don't be fooled into believing alcohol is an effective turn-on. A moderate amount reduces the inhibitions—but as Shakespeare said, it increases the desire but damages the performance.
—Ann Landers

I drink to forget I drink.
—Joe E. Lewis

Find out the brand of whiskey General Grant uses. I would like to furnish the same brand to my other generals.
—Abraham Lincoln on
complaints on Grant's
drinking

If you drink, don't drive. Don't even putt.
—Dean Martin

You think I'm an asshole now? You should have seen me when I was drunk.
—John Mellencamp

I sucked on a marijuana cigarette about a dozen times and once it did give me an orgasm that lasted three days. But then, I don't need pot, because my orgasms normally last that long anyway.
—Dudley Moore

I don't know, I never smoked Astroturf.
—Joe Namath on whether he
preferred grass or Astroturf

One more drink and I'll be under the host.
—Dorothy Parker

I feel sorry for people who don't drink, because when they get up in the morning, they're not going to feel any better all day.
—Frank Sinatra

An alcoholic is a man you don't like who drinks as much as you do.
—Dylan Thomas

Reality is a crutch for people who can't cope with drugs.
—Lily Tomlin

I don't have a drinking problem except when I can't get one.
—Tom Waits

Erogenous Zones

One of the great breakthroughs in sex has been the discovery of all the new erogenous zones. Once it was thought there were only a handful. Now they are all over the place, with new ones being reported every day.
—Bruce Jay Friedman

The fact is that there hasn't been a thrilling new erogenous zone discovered since de Sade.
—George Gilder

Erogenous zones are either everywhere or nowhere.
—Joseph Heller

Exhibitionism

Even though the labels "stripper" and "congressman" are completely incongruous, there was never anything but harmony in our hearts.
—Fanne Foxe on her
relationship with Wilbur Mills

49

I am a natural exhibitionist, and I get a thrill out of flashing my tits or, indeed, any other part of my body wherever possible.

—Xaviera Hollander

Don't see 'em this big out here, do they?

—Lyndon B. Johnson exposing himself to reporters in a public toilet when touring the Far East

It's not true that I had nothing on. I had on the radio.

—Marilyn Monroe on posing nude

I just look in the mirror and I say "God, it's really fantastic, the Lord really gave me something." So why on earth should I cover any of it up?

—Edy Williams

Fame

Of course, chicks keep popping up. When you're in a hotel, a pretty young lady makes life bearable.

—Roger Daltrey

The best thing about being famous is that it makes it easier to get laid.

—Allen Ginsberg

The naked little man tells the whole fucking world you're successful.

—Rock Hudson on the Oscar

I guess they like short blond women with big boobs.
—Dolly Parton on her
popularity in Japan

Winning a Grammy sure helped me get laid.
—Bonnie Raitt

Family Values

Mothers are fonder of their children because they are more certain they are their own.
—Aristotle

Everybody is trying to convince people that kids are interested in ecology, that kids are interested in politics. That's bullshit. Kids are interested in the same things that have always interested them: sex and violence.
—Alice Cooper

The first half of our lives is ruined by our parents and the second half by our children.
—Clarence Darrow

I come from a big family. As a matter of fact, I never got to sleep alone until I was married.
—Lewis Grizzard

Mom and Pop were just a couple of kids when they got married. He was eighteen, she was sixteen, and I was three.
—Billie Holiday

51

Literature is mostly about having sex and not much about having children. Life is the other way around.
—David Lodge

Look at the typical American family scene: Man walking around farting! Woman walking around scratching! Kids going around hollering, hey man, fuck that.
—Elvis Presley

If [a woman] is normally developed mentally, and well-bred, her sexual desire is small. If this were not so, the whole world would become a brothel and marriage and a family impossible.
—Dr. Joseph G. Richardson
(1909)

The greatest thing for any woman is to be a wife and mother.
—Theodore Roosevelt

I want to have children and I know my time is running out: I want to have them while my parents are still young enough to take care of them.
—Rita Rudner

In general, I support the conservative position and the family values movement. I don't see those people [Republicans] as gay bashers.
—John Schlafly, son of Phyllis,
when admitting he's gay

Biologically and temperamentally...women were made to be concerned first and foremost with childcare, husband care and homecare.
—Dr. Benjamin Spock

In my family sex was taboo. You don't screw anybody until you get married, you don't hold hands, you don't kiss, because you'll get a disease. It was all so awful that I had to develop a fantasy life.

—Barbra Streisand

Marriage was instituted by God himself for the purpose of preventing promiscuous intercourse of the sexes, for promoting domestic facility, and for securing the maintenance and security of children.

—Noah Webster

I have known more men destroyed by the desire to have wife and child and to keep them in comfort than I have seen destroyed by drink and harlots.

—William Butler Yeats

Fantasies

When turkeys mate, they think of swans.

—Johnny Carson

Sexual feelings for another person besides your spouse can be very strong...and very natural, but I'd keep it a fantasy if I were you and use it as a tool in your sex life with your wife.

—Marilyn Chambers

Oh stop, I want to feel my way along you, all over you and up and down you.

—Prince Charles to Camilla
Parker Bowles

What turns me on? Tuesday Weld in a dirty slip drinking beer.

—Alice Cooper

The last time I tried to make love with my wife nothing was happening so I said to her, "What's the matter, you can't think of anybody either?"

—Rodney Dangerfield

My husband said he wanted to have a relationship with a redhead so I dyed my hair red.

—Jane Fonda

If I had a cock for a day I would get myself pregnant.

—Germaine Greer

Men frequently fantasize fucking a nun, a nurse, or indeed a policewoman, and when I had my house, in New York, I had regular johns who would ask for girls in these various disguises.

—Xaviera Hollander

If your sexual fantasies were truly of interest to others, they would no longer be fantasies.

—Fran Lebowitz

During sex I fantasize that I'm someone else.

—Richard Lewis

Christ...Lincoln...Mimi Rogers.

—Rush Limbaugh on people
with whom he would share an
island

I'm aroused by the idea of a woman making love to me while either a man or another woman watches. Is that kinky?

—Madonna

Before I was famous, I had what you would call one-night stands. But I found these are much more exciting in my fantasies than in reality.

—John Travolta

Fantasy love is much better than reality love. Never doing it is very exciting. The most exciting attractions are between two opposites that never meet.

—Andy Warhol

What a man enjoys about a woman's clothes are his fantasies of how she would look without them.

—Evelyn Waugh

First Times

She stood up, looked at me appraisingly, then closed all the drapes. And I made love to Joan Crawford, or, rather she made love to me....She was all business....She would put me on her calendar for the next visit.

—Jackie Cooper

I was taught you had to be married to a man to sleep with him, so it wasn't until I was married the first time at twenty-six that I did it. God!

—Bette Davis

Then we got over into the back seat of the car, fumbling and feeling and scrambling for each other and I couldn't get it up.

—Bob Guccione

I lost my virginity, if you can call it that, when I was about thirteen. I think I was raped...she took it out and started gobbling.

—Liberace

I was crying and crying. When he started to spread my legs I went into a fit. I cried and screamed. I thought it was just a little thing and it stayed one size. I couldn't pee without hurting for a month.

—Loretta Lynn

I was so naive I didn't know where to put my peter. I was trying to put it in her belly button. After we finally did it, I felt so bad that I had sinned, I cried, I went to the Father and confessed.

—Billy Martin

The first girl you go to bed with is always pretty.

—Walter Matthau

Jesus, there's got to be more than this. If not, I'm going back to the other stuff because petting was a lot of fun.

—Victoria Principal

There wasn't any sensation for me, no orgasm or anything.

—Lou Rawls

I guess technically you can say I lost my virginity at age seven. I actually put it in her—a kid is practically born with a hard-on, you know.

—Bobby Riggs

Physically, it was like nothing. You read books, "She took to it like an animal." I just said, "Huh, is it over?" The whole thing lasted about a minute and a half, including buying the dress.

—Joan Rivers

Seduced and raped.

—George Bernard Shaw

I was horny and I enjoyed it a lot. Balling is always good, and sometimes it just knocks your brains out. The first time you ball somebody is always excellent.

—Grace Slick

I used to be goddamned well hung...losing my virginity didn't mean a damned thing to me. I thought dryfucking was actually more exciting. You know, just rubbing your prick against them until you came.

—Rudy Vallee

Flatulence

I should like one of these days to be so well known, so popular, so celebrated, so famous, that it would permit me to break wind in society, and society would think it a most natural thing.

—Honoré de Balzac

Farts are a repressed minority. The mouth gets to say all kinds of things, but the other place is supposed to keep quiet. But maybe our lower colons have something to say.
—Mel Brooks

In real life, people fart, right? But before *Blazing Saddles*, America had not come to terms with the fart.
—Mel Brooks

Cough and the world coughs with you. Fart and you stand alone.
—Trevor Griffiths

Fat dirty farts came shuttering out of your backside. You had an arse full of farts, darling, and I fucked them out of you, big fat fellows, long windy ones, quick little merry cracks.
—James Joyce

No, mind if I fart?
—Steve Martin when asked "Mind if I smoke?"

Did you ever fart in the catcher's face?
—Howard Stern in an interview with Ted Williams

I like to walk out of a restaurant with enough gas to open a Mobil station.
—Tom Waits

Gossip

First they say women like me too much, then they say women didn't like me at all, then they say that women like me too much again. Somewhere along the line they say that I secretly like men—but that men don't like me! I'm old, I'm young, I'm intelligent, I'm stupid. My tide goes in and out.

—Warren Beatty

If you told me Bill Clinton was very horny or very ambitious, I would have no trouble believing it. If you told me he was money hungry, I'd say that doesn't sound like the Bill Clinton I know.

—David Broder

I admire Ted Kennedy. How many fifty-nine-year-olds still go to Florida for spring vacation?

—Pat Buchanan

A good housekeeper but a whore at heart.

—Butch Cassidy on Etta Place

What do you expect. She sleeps with the boss.

—Joan Crawford on actress
Norma Shearer

She's the original good time that was had by all.

—Bette Davis on a rival actress

Bill Clinton has a small penis and Hillary has broad ankles.

—Gennifer Flowers

...slept with everybody to get to the top.

—La Toya Jackson on Madonna

Mick screws many but has few affairs.

—Bianca Jagger on her ex-
husband Mick

She'd never have a nooner with anyone—she'd never mess up her hair in the middle of the day.

—Kitty Kelley on Nancy Reagan
(paraphrasing Nancy's
hairdresser)

Am I cynical, or does anyone else think the only reason Warren Beatty decided to have a child is so that he can meet babysitters?

—David Letterman

I bet he doesn't put his hand up her dress.

—Marilyn Monroe on JFK's
relationship with Jackie
Kennedy

The worst thing I've heard about the Kennedys is that they're very smart but when they get horny, their penis takes over and their brain closes.

—Florence Orbach

A vacuum with nipples.

—Otto Preminger on Marilyn
Monroe

So what's the big deal. The kid's not even related to him.
—Gary Shandling quoting Jerry
Lee Lewis on Michael Jackson

Health

I'm probably the only model in New York who hasn't had breast implants.
—Kim Alexis

The only reason I would take up jogging is so that I could hear heavy breathing again.
—Erma Bombeck

My breast operations were a nightmare. They were really botched in every way.
—Cher

And there is definitely life after oat bran. All our nation has to show after years of that is diarrhea.
—Julia Child

After two days in the hospital, I took a turn for the nurse.
—W. C. Fields

I think making love is the best form of exercise.
—Cary Grant

Sexual exercise can do a lot for your penis...Practice sometimes makes perfect and can increase the size of a student pecker.
—Xaviera Hollander

I don't know of a better exercise for keeping a man's sexual apparatus in good shape than having regular sex, either by getting sucked, fucked, or in case of an emergency, by masturbation.

—Xaviera Hollander

Love can be terribly obscene. It is love that causes the neuroticism of the day. It is love that is the prime cause of tuberculosis.

—D. H. Lawrence

I don't need a psychiatrist, I need a man.

—Marilyn Monroe.

If I don't do it everyday, I get a headache.

—Willie Nelson

Only time can heal a broken heart, just as only time can heal his broken arms and legs.

—Miss Piggy

Homophobia

Whatever war you were in, I know it was before the Clinton fags-in-the-foxhole [proposal].

—Warren Barry

Two men necking, lying in bed...get an automatic or an Uzi instead. Shoot them now.

—Buju Bauton

I hate homosexuals; I pray for them.

—Anita Bryant

I don't hate homosexuals. I love homosexuals. It's the sin of homosexuality I hate.

—Anita Bryant

If homosexuality were the normal way, God would have made Adam and Bruce.

—Anita Bryant

As a mother, I know that homosexuals cannot biologically reproduce children; therefore, they must recruit our children.

—Anita Bryant

We're well aware of the male homosexual problem in this country, which is of course minor, but to our certain knowledge there is not one lesbian in England.

—Lord Chamberlain

What can you say about a country that tolerates homosexuals but not smokers? I never gave anyone AIDS.

—Tom Clancy

Homosexuality is a sickness, just as are baby rape or wanting to become head of General Motors.

—Eldridge Cleaver

It is a great injustice to persecute homosexuality as a crime, and a cruelty too.

—Sigmund Freud

The party of homosexuals.

—Orrin Hatch on the
Democratic party

Movies were anti-gay. Movies are anti-gay. And movies will continue to be anti-gay.

—Rock Hudson

There is probably no sensitive heterosexual alive who is not preoccupied with his latent homosexuality.

—Norman Mailer

Homosexuality itself is not against the law, just practicing it is.

—Anthony Mancini

I am rather tired of democracy being made safe for the pimps and prostitutes, the spivs and pansies, and now the queers.

—Sir Cyril Osborne

A very positive message.

—Dan Quayle on a church sermon condemning homosexuality as satanic

If I'm in the shower, I like to know that I'm not being ogled over by some guy.

—Mike Tuttle, GI, on gays in the military

If you say a homosexual is a crippled personality, who can blame him? All his life he's heard that he's a sick, perverted, abominable, loathsome creature or some kind of a freak. He's had to live like a criminal much of the time.

—Abigail Van Buren

Homosexuality, Female

What's the point of being a lesbian if a woman is going to look and act like an imitation man?
—Rita Mae Brown

Martina was so far in the closet she was in danger of being a garment bag.
—Rita Mae Brown on her relationship with Martina Navratilova

I don't want to go to jail because I'm afraid of lesbians.
—Zsa Zsa Gabor

All women are lesbians, except those who don't know it yet.
—Jill Johnson

A woman lover is always persistant.
—Hedy Lamarr

Girls who put out are tramps. Girls who don't are ladies....Should one of you boys happen upon a girl who doesn't put out, do not jump to the conclusion that you have found a lady. What you have probably found is a lesbian.
—Fran Lebowitz

Many years ago I chased a woman for almost two years, only to discover her tastes were exactly like mine: we were both crazy about girls.
—Groucho Marx

Seventy-five per cent of our time at least is spent on lesbians.

—William Masters

Dad and I had breakfast this morning. We had a look at each other's speeches. He would have used mine, but he's not a lesbian. I would have used his, but I'm not a Republican.

—Diane Mosbacher, daughter of
Commerce Secretary Robert
Mosbacher, under George
Bush

I get hit on all the time by gay women. I'm flattered that they like me… but I'm not gay.

—Dolly Parton

One vagina plus another vagina equals zero.

—Dr. David Reuben

Oh! I want to put my arms around you. I ache to hold you close. Your ring is a great comfort. I look at it and think she does love me or I wouldn't be wearing it.

—Eleanor Roosevelt in a letter
to her lover Lorena Hickcock

The hell with you, bitch. I got twelve women on this show and I can have one every night if I want.

—Kate Smith

I love women…. If I could get into it, it would be great. But you know, it don't mean a thing if it ain't got that schwing!

—Sharon Stone on whether she
has had sex with a woman

I am not a lesbian and I am not a slut.
—Vanessa Williams

Homosexuality, General

We need laws that protect everyone. Men and women, straights and gays, regardless of sexual perversion... uh, persuasion.
—Bella Abzug

The love that previously dared not speak its name has now grown hoarse from screaming it.
—Robert Brustein

You don't need to be straight to fight and die for your country. You just need to shoot straight.
—Barry Goldwater

Homosexuals work at sex more. They invest of themselves and probably get a little more back.
—Virginia Johnson

We have never treated homosexuality as a disease or defined it to a patient as a handicap.
—Masters and Johnson

Psychology and psychiatry have abandoned a whole population of people who feel dissatisfied with homosexuality.
—Joseph Nicolosi

"Gay" used to be one of the most agreeable words in the language. Its appropriation by a notably morose group is an act of piracy.
—Arthur Schlesinger Jr.

Have I lived an alternate lifestyle? The answer is no.
—Donna Shalala on whether
she is gay

The main thing is that the act male homosexuals commit is ugly and repugnant and afterwards they are disgusted with themselves. They drink and take drugs....In women it is the opposite. They do nothing that they are disgusted by.
—Gertrude Stein

The homosexual subculture based on brief, barren assignations is, in part, a dark mirror of the sex-obsessed majority culture.
—George Will

Homosexuality, Male

Perhaps most actors are latent homosexuals and we cover it up with drink. I was once a homosexual, but it didn't work.
—Richard Burton

I hadn't been in prep school more than a month, and I'd slept with all the boys and half the faculty. Of course, I'm speaking rhetorically.
—Truman Capote

I'm an alcoholic, I'm a drug addict. I'm a homosexual. I'm a genius.

> —Truman Capote

I've been turned down for everything, including the WACs.

> —Truman Capote on his
> rejection from the draft

Killer fruit.

> —Truman Capote describing J.
> Edgar Hoover

...falls in love passionately with air-conditioning repairmen.

> —Gore Vidal on Truman Capote

The majority of those men are homosexual—perhaps not the majority—but in the USA there are already twenty-five percent of them and in England and Germany it is the same. You cannot imagine it in the history of France.

> —Edith Cresson

I've had my cock sucked by five of the big names in Hollywood. I wanted more than anything to get some little part.

> —James Dean

People think heteros make love and gays have sex. I want to tell them that's wrong.

> —Boy George

People already think I'm that way—homo—because of my voice, and I'm not.

> —Michael Jackson

Homosexuals make the best friends because they care about you as a woman and are not jealous. They love you but don't try to screw up your head.

—Bianca Jagger

Ten percent of all men are, more or less, exclusively homosexual for at least three years between the ages of sixteen and fifty-five.

—Alfred Kinsey

Long-term relationships between two males are notably few.

—Alfred Kinsey

Homosexuals do not normally follow men who offer dicks that appear to be no bigger than ziti macaroni.

—Reverend Boyd McDonald

I appreciate Representative Frank trying to enhance my dull image, but in terms of obsession with sex, I'm not in Barney's league.

—Senator Sam Nunn

Most of my male friends are gay, and that seems perfectly natural to me. I mean, who wouldn't like cock?

—Valerie Perrine

Boy George is all England needs—another queen who can't dress.

—Joan Rivers

If you talk about sex three times in the same evening, a girl will refer to you as an animal. But if a homosexual talks about it all day, that's fine, because that is his craft.

—Mort Sahl

Before *Shampoo* [the movie] we hairdressers were queens, now we're machos. In truth, we are neither.
—Vidal Sassoon

Homosexuals are crazy about me because I'm so flamboyant. They love to imitate the things I say and the way I act, and they like the way I move my body.
—Mae West

I have to feel sad for all the thousands of women who fantasized about being in his arms, who now have to realize that he never really cared about them. I heard one woman say, "I used to dream about him; too bad he really didn't like erotic relations with women."
—Dr. Ruth Westheimer on Rock Hudson

Horniness

So many women and so little time.
—John Barrymore

Oh God. I'll just live inside your trousers or something.
—Prince Charles in a phone conversation with Camilla Parker Bowles

The big mistake that men make is that when they've reached puberty, they believe that they like women. Actually, you're just horny.
—Jules Feiffer

This attractive lady whom I had only recently been introduced to dropped into my lap....I chose not to dump her off.

—Gary Hart on Donna Rice

When you are really ripe for a girl you always get one. You did not have to think about it. Sooner or later it would come.

—Ernest Hemingway

Ten days of abstinence awakens passion.

—Ricardo Montalban

Tell him I've been too fucking busy—or vice versa.

—Dorothy Parker

I can always be distracted by love, but eventually I get horny for my creativity.

—Gilda Radner

When you are a young you always assume that sex was invented the day you hit puberty.

—John P. Roche

If you have any doubts as to virility, dismiss them from your mind. I was not impotent, I was not sterile. I was not homosexual and I was extremely, though not promiscuously, susceptible.

—George Bernard Shaw

Ideal Partner

I'm not that finicky.... But I'll tell you this, I'll work with any son of a bitch, but I won't sleep with a bitch.
—Mikhail Baryshnikov

I'd marry again if I found a man who had $15 million and would sign over half of it to me before the marriage, and guarantee he'd be dead within a year.
—Bette Davis

I want a man who's kind and understanding. Is that too much to ask of a millionaire?
—Zsa Zsa Gabor

A woman must be a cute, cuddly, naive little thing—tender, sweet, and stupid.
—Adolf Hitler

Throughout history, females have picked providers for mates. Males have picked anything.
—Margaret Mead

Your traditional well-built woman, meaning large breasts, small waist, good butt, good legs. That's my sexual ideal.
—John Travolta

Impotence/Frigidity

Men always fall for frigid women, because they put on the best show.
—Fanny Brice

When his cock wouldn't stand up he blew his head off. He sold himself a line of bullshit and he bought it.
—Germaine Greer on Ernest Hemingway

When I hear his steps outside my door I lie down on my bed, close my eyes, open my legs and think of England.
—Lady Alice Hillingdon (1912)

Though a man may be a dignified judge, a captain of industry, a national golf champion, or a distinguished physicist, he feels worthless and debased if he cannot perform an act which he shares in common with dogs, rabbits, cattle, and rats.
—Howard R. and Martha E. Lewis

A woman's a woman until the day she dies, but a man's only a man as long as he can.
—Moms Mabley

I'm scared to death of the individual who has no sexual desires, no romantic desires, no fantasies.
—John Cardinal O'Connor

Impotence is a penis that won't do what it's told.
—Dr. David Reuben

Infatuation

I have a sexual crush on Brigitte Bardot. It's purely sex. I've never seen one of her movies. It would destroy me. I've seen her still photographs. I find her so devastating that if I ever saw her moving around I would probably kill myself.
—Woody Allen

Absolutely pure animal magnetism. Suddenly there was just the two of us. Everyone else melted away.
—Tipper Gore describing her meeting with husband Al

Don't you think we could have a beautiful chocolate-covered daughter together?
—Margaret Trudeau on Lou Rawls

Is that a gun in your pocket, or are you just glad to see me?
—Mae West

Infidelity/Adultery

It is better to be unfaithful than to be faithful without wanting to be.
—Brigitte Bardot

Fidelity, *n*. A virtue peculiar to those who are about to be betrayed.

—Ambrose Bierce

My mother-in-law broke up my marriage. One day my wife came home early from work and found us in bed together.

—Lenny Bruce

Why doesn't anybody ask if I've had an affair?

—Barbara Bush when asked
about her husband's private
life

I have looked on a lot of women with lust. I've committed adultry in my heart many times.

—Jimmy Carter

Christ says, don't consider yourself better than someone else because one guy screws a whole bunch of women while the other guy is loyal to his wife.

—Jimmy Carter

I told my wife the truth. I told her I was seeing a psychiatrist. Then she told me the truth: that she was seeing a psychiatrist, two plumbers, and a bartender.

—Rodney Dangerfield

In Europe, extramarital affairs are considered a sign of good health, a feat.

—Jean-Pierre Detremerie on Bill
Clinton's alleged affairs

The more beautiful the single red rose he brings you, the more gorgeous the tramp he's fooling around with.

—Phyllis Diller

The chain of wedlock is so heavy that it takes two to carry it—sometimes three.
—Alexandre Dumas

I say I don't sleep with married men, but what I mean is I don't sleep with happily married men.
—Britt Ekland

Adultery can be a more "healthy" recreation than, for example, the game of mah-jongg or watching television.
—Dr. Albert Ellis

I feel I'm the person responsible for putting Bill Clinton in the White House.
—Gennifer Flowers on the publicity created by her allegations she had an affair with Clinton

I gave Bill a huge piece of my heart for many, many years. Now it appears the man I loved...was cheating on me too. Left and right.
—Gennifer Flowers on Clinton

How many husbands have I had? You mean apart from my own?
—Zsa Zsa Gabor

If my wife cheated, I'd kill her. She's part of my property. I feel I own her, the way I own my car, and I don't lend my car out to people.
—Al Goldstein

Women feel dirty, men don't.
—Jerry Hall on sex without love

The world wants to be cheated. So cheat!
—Xaviera Hollander

Remember the old proverb: It is no use crying over spilt milk—or sperm.
—Xaviera Hollander

We women tend to be insecure creatures, and if our husbands or lovers can't get it up, our immediate instinct is to accuse him of screwing someone else.
—Xaviera Hollander

If a woman hasn't got a tiny streak of harlot in her, she's as dry as a stick as a rule.
—D. H. Lawrence

Sammy Davis Jr. had his own code of marital fidelity. He explained to me that he could do anything with me except have normal intercourse because that would be cheating on his wife.
—Linda Lovelace

There's nothing like a good dose of another woman to make a man appreciate his wife.
—Claire Booth Luce

My attitude toward men who mess around is simple: If you find them, kill them.
—Loretta Lynn

There is one thing I would break up over, and that is if she caught me with another woman. I won't stand for that.
—Steve Martin

We in the industry know that behind every successful screenwriter stands a woman. And behind her stands his wife.

—Groucho Marx

Some people claim that marriage interferes with romance. There's no doubt about it. Anytime you have a romance, your wife is bound to interfere.

—Groucho Marx

There's nothing more disgusting than a person who would commit adultery! You swore fidelity...your life is involved with a marriage partner. Who the hell are you to cheat on her?

—Jackie Mason

When a man brings his wife flowers for no reason—there's a reason.

—Molly McGee

Adultery is the application of democracy to love.

—H. L. Mencken

Husbands are chiefly good lovers when they are betraying their wives.

—Marilyn Monroe

I am too interested in other men's wives to think about getting one of my own.

—George Moore

I don't think there are any men who are faithful to their wives.

—Jackie Kennedy Onassis

He and I had an office so tiny that an inch smaller and it would have been adultery.

—Dorothy Parker

I enjoy dating married men because they don't want anything kinky, like breakfast.

—Joan Rivers

It's hard to maintain a one-on-one relationship if the other person is not going to allow me to be with other people.

—Axl Rose

I finally found a broad I can cheat on.

—Frank Sinatra on new wife
Mia Farrow

My wife doesn't care what I do when I'm away as long as I don't have a good time.

—Lee Trevino

Young men want to be faithful, and are not; old men want to be faithless, and cannot.

—Oscar Wilde

Next to the pleasure of making a new mistress is that of being rid of an old one.

—William Wycherley

Jealousy

Each [of my wives] was jealous and resentful of my preoccupation with business. Yet none showed any visible aversion to sharing the proceeds.

—J. Paul Getty

Jealousy is the fear of losing the thing you love most. It's very normal. Suspicion is the thing that's abnormal.
—Jerry Hall

Jewelry

A lovely ring that I wear in a very special place. One of my [vaginal] lips...it's pierced, and he thought that this part of my body had made a lot of money and fame and it deserved a present.
—Marilyn Chambers on a gift bought for her by Sammy Davis Jr.

I never hated a man enough to give back his diamonds.
—Zsa Zsa Gabor

A diamond is the only kind of ice that keeps a girl warm.
—Elizabeth Taylor

I have a lust for diamonds, almost like a disease.
—Elizabeth Taylor

Kinky Behavior

Is sex dirty? Only if it's done right.
—Woody Allen

The requirements of romantic love are difficult to satisfy in the trunk of a Dodge Dart.
—Lisa Alther

It can be great fun to have an affair with a bitch.
—Louis Auchincloss

I've tried several varieties of sex. The conventional position makes me claustrophobic, and the others either give me a stiff neck or lockjaw.
—Tallulah Bankhead

I can't get aroused until I see a pair of rubber dice hanging from the mirror.
—Johnny Carson

Maybe I'll make a *Mary Poppins* movie and shove the umbrella up my ass.
—Marilyn Chambers

In Washington getting laid is considered kinky sex.
—Nancy Collins

She was so wild, when she made French toast she got her tongue caught in the toaster.
—Rodney Dangerfield

If it weren't for pickpockets, I'd have no love life at all.
—Rodney Dangerfield

My mother didn't breastfeed me. She said she liked me as a friend.
—Rodney Dangerfield

Ever since the young men have owned motorcycles, incest has been dying out.
—Max Frisch

I understand women. All I know is women. I'm surprised I didn't grow up to be a transvestite.

—Arsenio Hall

I would go to seedy places in the New York area and dance on tables, with drunken men whipping out their hoo-has.

—Goldie Hawn

I saw a young couple against the wall. The boy was urinating against the wall and the girl never let go of his arm. She'd look down at what he was doing, then look around at the scenery, then back at the boy. I felt this was true love at work.

—Alfred Hitchcock

I'd rather laugh in bed than do it.... If I went to a lady of the night, I'd probably pay her to tell me jokes. Would that be perverted?

—Billy Joel

Many, many people have done a lot more sexual experimentation than I have. Yet it's the one who writes about it who is thought to be weird.

—Erica Jong

The trouble with incest is that it gets you involved with relatives.

—George S. Kaufman

Recently I had this crazy, passionate thing with a guy who wants to make love in parking lots and telephone booths. Just great. But fidelity is a problem for me.

—Margot Kidder

There's photographs of me groveling about, crawling about Amsterdam on my knees, coming out of whorehouses and things like that.

—John Lennon

It's very dangerous to stick it up a woman's ass. It tends to make them more promiscuous...because she's doing her best to be faithful to that dull pup she's got for a man, and she knows if it blasts into the center of her stubbornness, that's the end....She won't be able to hold on to fidelity.

—Norman Mailer

My husband is German; every night I get dressed up like Poland and he invades me.

—Bette Midler

It's been so long since I made love, I can't remember who gets tied up.

—Joan Rivers

Before we make love, my husband takes a painkiller.

—Joan Rivers

He had a red dress on, and a black feather boa around his neck....And Hoover had a Bible. He wanted one of the boys to read from the Bible. And he read...and the other boy played with him, wearing the rubber gloves.

—Susan Rosenstiel quoted in
*Official and Confidential: The
Secret Life of J. Edgar Hoover*

The closest I ever came to a menage à trois was once I dated a schizophrenic.

—Rita Rudner

Human beings are infinitely adaptable. If they can do it in the back seat of a '57 Chevy, they can do it anywhere.
—Dr. Patricia Santy on sex in
space

I'm not kinky, but occasionally I like to put on a robe and stand in front of a tennis ball machine.
—Gary Shandling

Streaking. Mooning. Ballwalking. Leg Shaving. Belly/Navel Shots. Chicken Fights. Butt Biting.
—Chapter titles in the
Pentagon's report on the 1991
Tailhook Association
convention

Who has put that pubic hair on my Coke?
—Clarence Thomas according
to Anita Hill

She said he proposed something on their wedding night her own brother wouldn't have suggested.
—James Thurber

Very few people will suck toes. They think it is foot fetishism. People don't want to suck toes and they don't want to talk about life. Men always expect you to suck them but they don't suck.
—Lily Tomlin

He said he was going to lick me all over.

> —Congressional aide Kari
> Tupper on what Senator Brock
> Adams told her

Kissing

I married the first man I ever kissed. When I tell my children that, they just about throw up.

> —Barbara Bush

It's like kissing Hitler.

> —Tony Curtis on Marilyn
> Monroe

The kiss originated when the first male reptile licked the first female reptile, implying in a subtle, complimentary way that she is as succulent as the small reptile he had for dinner the night before.

> —F. Scott Fitzgerald

It's the kissiest business in the world. You have to keep kissing people.

> —Ava Gardner on the film
> industry

Never delay kissing a pretty girl or opening a bottle of whiskey.

> —Ernest Hemingway

People who throw kisses are hopelessly lazy.

> —Bob Hope

A genuine kiss generates so much heat it destroys germs.
—Dr. S. L. Katzoff (1940)

I wasn't kissing her. I was whispering in her mouth.
—Chico Marx

When women kiss it always reminds me of prizefighters shaking hands.
—H. L. Mencken

Blondes have the hottest kisses. Redheads are fair to middling torrid, and brunettes are the frigidest of all. It's something to do with hormones, no doubt.
—Ronald Reagan

Were kisses all the joys in bed, one woman would another wed.
—William Shakespeare

I kissed my first woman and smoked my first cigarette on the same day. I haven't had time for tobacco since.
—Arturo Toscanini

I can't give too many kisses. The press is watching. Perhaps later.
—Pierre Trudeau to a female campaign worker

Two people kissing always look like fish.
—Andy Warhol

Everybody winds up kissing the wrong person good night.
—Andy Warhol

Few men know how to kiss well; fortunately, I've always had time to teach them.

—Mae West

Love

The difference between sex and love is that sex relieves tension and love causes it.

—Woody Allen

Love is the answer, but while you are waiting for the answer, sex raises some pretty good questions.

—Woody Allen

Sensual enjoyment without a union of souls is bestial and will always remain bestial; after it one experiences not a trace of noble sentiment, but rather regret.

—Ludwig van Beethoven

Love, *n*. A temporary insanity curable by marriage.

—Ambrose Bierce

I have never loved anyone for love's sake, except perhaps, Josephine—a little.

—Napoleon Bonaparte

Like the measles, love is most dangerous when it comes late in life.

—Lord Byron

Lust isn't all there is to sex. Sex isn't all there is to love. But love is almost all there is to life.

—Eddie Cantor

I would never make it with some guy I'd just met...Sex is a dumb thing unless you love somebody.
—Cher

Many a man has fallen in love with a girl in light so dim he would not have chosen a suit by it.
—Maurice Chevalier

Love is a fire. But whether it is going to warm your heart or burn down your house, you can never tell.
—Joan Crawford

I love Mickey Mouse more than any woman I've ever known.
—Walt Disney

Love without esteem cannot go far or reach high. It is an angel with only one wing.
—Alexandre Dumas

Love is indescribable and unconditional: I could tell you a thousand things it is not, but not one thing that it is.
—Duke Ellington

Where they love they do not desire and where they desire they do not love.
—Sigmund Freud

Sexual love is undoubtably one of the chief things in life. Apart from a few queers, all the world knows this.
—Sigmund Freud

One is very crazy when in love.
—Sigmund Freud

There is hardly any activity, any enterprise, which is started with such tremendous hopes and expectations and yet which fails so regularly as love.

—Erich Fromm

It's an extra dividend when you like the girl you're in love with.

—Clark Gable

Love is the self-delusion we manufacture to justify the trouble we take to have sex.

—Dan Greenburg

The drug which makes sexuality palatable in popular mythology.

—Germaine Greer

Unless there's some emotional tie, I'd rather play tennis.

—Bianca Jagger

Love has no great influence upon the sum of life.

—Samuel Johnson

As for that topsy-turvy known as soixante-neuf, personally I have always felt it to be madly confusing, like trying to pat your head and rub your tummy at the same time.

—Helen Lawrenson

Love is only the dirty trick played on us to achieve continuation of the species.

—W. Somerset Maugham

Love is like war: easy to begin but very hard to stop.

—H. L. Mencken

Love is not the dying moan of a violin—it's the triumphant twang of a bedspring.

> —S. J. Perelman

Love is a grave mental disease.

> —Plato

Love will never be ideal until man recovers from the illusion that he can be just a little bit faithful or a little bit married.

> —Helen Rowland

Before I met my husband, I'd never fallen in love, though I'd stepped in it a few times.

> —Rita Rudner

Love is a wonderful thing, but as long as it is blind, I will never be out of a job.

> —Justice Selby, a divorce court judge

Love is blind.

> —William Shakespeare

All's fair in love and war.

> —F. E. Smedley

To me love is being able to go to bed with someone and feel better about them when you wake up the next morning.

> —Sylvester Stallone

Some women and men seem to need each other.

> —Gloria Steinem

'Tis better to have loved and lost, than never to have loved at all.

—Tennyson

There is no remedy for love but to love more.

—Henry David Thoreau

If love is the answer, could you rephrase the question?

—Lily Tomlin

Love is the same as like except you feel sexier. And also more annoyed when he talks with his mouth full. And you also resent it more when he interrupts you. And you also respect him less when he shows any weakness. And furthermore, when you ask him to pick you up at the airport and he tells you he can't do it because he's busy, it's only when you love him that you hate him.

—Judith Viorst

I never loved another person the way I love myself.

—Mae West

Love conquers all things except poverty and toothache.

—Mae West

To love oneself is the beginning of a lifelong romance.

—Oscar Wilde

Just another four-letter word.

—Tennessee Williams

Platonic love is from the neck up.
                                    —Thyra Winslow

Male Chauvinism

Nature intended women to be our slaves...they are our
property; we are not theirs....What a mad idea to
demand equality for women! Women are nothing but
machines for producing children.
                                    —Napoleon Bonaparte

Everybody makes me out to be some kind of a macho pig,
humping women in the gutter. I do, but I put a pillow
under them first.
                                    —James Caan

The only position for women in the SNCC is prone.
                                    —Stokely Carmichael

Every woman needs a man to discover her.
                                    —Charlie Chaplin

You only had one thing that wasn't terrible, and that was
the thing between your legs. It didn't take you long to
make the most of that one talent. I have as much interest
in touching you as I'd have in making love to Attila the
Hun.
                                    —Charlie Chaplin to his
                                    pregnant lover

There is a kind of Neanderthal swing back to tits and
ass....It's different today than in the seventies, when we
had the feminist reaction. We've slid back.
                                    —Devorah Cutter on Hollywood

Of all the criminals on the earth, none is so brutish as man when he seeks the delirium of coition.
—Edward Dahlberg

Men want women they can turn on and off like a light switch.
—Ian Fleming

We've been castrated. It's all very well to let a bullock out into the field when you've already cut off his balls because you know he's not going to do anything. That's exactly what's happened to women.
—Germaine Greer

All they can see when they look at me is my breasts; I have a brain too.
—Jean Harlow

Women's libbers are a pain in the ass.
—Evel Knievel

Man is willing to accept woman as an equal, as a man in skirts, as an angel, a devil, a baby face, a bosom, a womb, a pair of legs...an ideal or an obscenity: the only thing he won't accept her as is a human being, a real human being of the female sex.
—D. H. Lawrence

Women should be obscene not heard.
—Groucho Marx

When a woman becomes a scholar, there is usually something wrong with her sexual organs.
—Friedrich Nietzsche

Hunt, pursue, and capture are biologically programmed into the male sexuality.
—Camille Paglia

For a guy part of the ego trip is being able to satisfy women. You like each one to tell you you're the greatest lay they ever had...and the really smart women, they give you that and tell you that you are.
—Bobby Riggs

I watch George Carlin, who's brilliant, and every other word is "fuck," "piss," "suck," and nobody says this man is dirty. I walk on stage and say one "fuck" and the whole review the next day is dedicated to this filthy woman.
—Joan Rivers

A woman's place is in the stove.
—Mort Sahl

It is a gentlemen's first duty to remember in the morning who it was he took to bed with him.
—Dorothy L. Sayers

It is a natural law of man to go after women, even married women. Of course, it may be true that he has little respect for them after. But why bother your head about that? There's something else. Women who are unfaithful should be shot.
—Pancho Villa

Women have the right to work, as long as they have dinner ready when you get home.
—John Wayne

The only way to behave to a woman is to make love to her, if she is pretty, and to someone else, if she is not.
—Oscar Wilde

When a man is seen with a lot of women, it's "Oh, which one did he grace?" But if a woman is seen with a lot of men, she's just a slut.
—Debra Winger

Marriage

When two people marry they become, in the eyes of the law, one person, and that one person is the husband.
—Shana Alexander

I tended to place my wife under a pedestal.
—Woody Allen

Many a man owes his success to his first wife and his second wife to his success.
—Jim Backus

To marry while blindly in love is dangerous; to marry without it may be fatal.
—Brigitte Bardot

The other night I said to my wife, Ruth, "Do you feel that the sex and excitement has gone out of our marriage?" Ruth said, "I'll discuss it with you during the next commercial."
—Milton Berle

Marriage, *n*. The state or condition of a community consisting of a master, a mistress, and two slaves, making in all, two.

—Ambrose Bierce

I wonder if the fucking you get is worth the fucking you get.

—Humphrey Bogart on his
fourth marriage

Marriage is not just spiritual communion and passionate embraces; marriage is also three meals a day and remembering to carry out the trash.

—Dr. Joyce Brothers

Marriage—the longing for the deep, deep peace of the double bed after the hurly-burly of the chaise longue.

—Mrs. Patrick Campbell

The trouble with some women is that they get all excited about nothing; and then they marry him.

—Cher

What do I know of sex? I'm a married man.

—Tom Clancy

The most happy marriage I can picture...would be the union of a deaf man to a blind woman.

—Samuel Taylor Coleridge

I never married because I have three pets at home that answer the same purpose as a husband. I have a dog that growls every morning, a parrot that swears all afternoon, and a cat that comes home late at night.

—Marie Corelli

We sleep in separate bedrooms, we have dinner apart, we take separate vacations—we're doing everything we can to keep our marriage together.

—Rodney Dangerfield

The man, my dear, is never going to make a marriage work. If it works, the woman does it.

—Bette Davis

Every woman should marry—and no man.

—Benjamin Disraeli

Any intelligent woman who reads the marriage contract and then goes into it deserves all the consequences.

—Isadora Duncan

We were happily married for eight months. Unfortunately we were married for four and a half years.

—Nick Faldo

Keep your eyes wide open before marriage and half shut afterwards.

—Benjamin Franklin

It's never easy keeping your own husband happy. It's much easier to make someone else's husband happy.

—Zsa Zsa Gabor

Husbands are like fires—they go out when unattended.

—Zsa Zsa Gabor

A man is incomplete until he is married. Then he is finished.

—Zsa Zsa Gabor

I know nothing about sex, because I was always married.
—Zsa Zsa Gabor

I like the teacher-student aspects.
—Hugh Hefner on his marriage
to a much younger woman

Matrimony—the high sea for which no compass has yet been invented.
—Heinrich Heine

...great for taxes, necessary for children, but abominable for romance.
—Lauren Hutton

The French rule is wise, that no lady dances after marriage. This is founded in solid physical reasons, gestation and nursing leaving little time to a married lady when this exercise can be either safe or innocent.
—Thomas Jefferson

Second marriage: the triumph of hope over experience.
—Samuel Johnson

Marriage has many pains, but celibacy has no pleasures.
—Samuel Johnson

My favorite hobby? I married them all.
—Stan Laurel

The honeymoon is over when he phones to say he'll be late for supper and she's already left a note that it's in the refrigerator.
—Bill Lawrence

Marriage is neither heaven or hell. It is simply purgatory.
—Abraham Lincoln

I belong to Bridegrooms Anonymous. Whenever I feel like getting married, they send over a lady in a housecoat and hair curlers to burn my toast.
—Dick Martin

Politics doesn't make strange bedfellows—marriage does.
—Groucho Marx

The first relationship is for sex; the second is for children; the third is for companionship.
—Margaret Mead

The only really happy people are married women and single men.
—H. L. Mencken

Marriage is the alliance of two people, one who never remembers birthdays and the other who never forgets them.
—Ogden Nash

If there is a realistic deterrent to marriage it's the fact that you can't afford divorce.
—Jack Nicholson

When a girl marries she exchanges the attention of many men for the inattention of one.
—Helen Rowland

Before marriage, a man declares that he would lay down his life to serve you; after marriage, he won't even lay down his newspaper to talk to you.

—Helen Rowland

A husband is what is left after the lover has been extracted.

—Helen Rowland

A marriage is likely to be called happy if neither party ever expected to get much happiness out of it.

—Bertrand Russell

When two people are under the influence of the most violent, most insane, most delusive and most transient of passions, they are required to swear that they will remain in that excited, abnormal, and exhausting condition continuously until death do them part.

—George Bernard Shaw

A man has no business to marry a woman who can't make him miserable. It means she can't make him happy.

—George Bernard Shaw

Marriage is popular because it combines the maximum of temptation with the maximum of opportunity.

—George Bernard Shaw

There is never any real sex in romance; what is more, there is very little, and that of a very crude kind, in ninety-nine hundredths of our married life.

—George Bernard Shaw

I'd like to get married because I like the idea of a man being required by law to sleep with me every night.
—Carrie Snow

By all means marry; if you get a good wife, you'll be happy. If you get a bad one, you'll become a philosopher.
—Socrates

Marriage: a ceremony in which rings are put on the finger of the lady and through the nose of the gentleman.
—Herbert Spencer

Some of us are becoming the men we wanted to marry.
—Gloria Steinem

The reason why so few marriages are happy is because young ladies spend their time in making nets, not making cages.
—Jonathan Swift

A successful man is one who makes more money than his wife can spend. A successful woman is one who can find such a man.
—Lana Turner

In biblical times a man could have as many wives as he could afford. Just like today.
—Abigail Van Buren

I've married a few people I shouldn't have, but haven't we all?
—Mamie Van Doren

Marriage is a great institution, but I'm not ready for an institution yet.
—Mae West

If they could come to my office, I really do believe I could help them.
—Dr. Ruth Westheimer on the marital problems of Prince Charles and Princess Diana

One should always be in love. That is the reason one should never marry.
—Oscar Wilde

The one charm of marriage is that it makes a life of deception absolutely necessary for both parties.
—Oscar Wilde

Whenever you want to marry someone, go have lunch with his ex-wife.
—Shelley Winters

I did a picture in England one winter and it was so cold I almost got married.
—Shelley Winters

Masturbation

Don't knock masturbation. It's sex with someone you love.
—Woody Allen

I was the best I ever had.
—Woody Allen

The good thing about masturbation is that you don't have to dress up for it.

—Truman Capote

When the practice is begun at an early age, both mental and physical development may be notably interfered with. It is often stated that masturbation is a cause of insanity, epilepsy, and hysteria. I believe it to be more likely that the masturbation is the first manifestation of a developing insanity.

—Dr. Charles Hunter Dunn
(1920)

I recommend masturbation because it's cheaper and you meet a better class of people that way.

—Buddy Hackett

Sex without love is just two people masturbating together.

—John Holmes

Masturbation! The amazing availability of it!

—James Joyce

A woman occasionally is quite a serviceable substitute for masturbation.

—Karl Kraus

The first time I masturbated...it flew across the room and hit the far wall.

—Jack Lemmon

Masturbation is always safe, because there you not only control the person you're with, but you can leave when you want to.

—Dudley Moore

No minister, moralist, teacher, or scientific researcher has ever shown any evidence that masturbation is harmful in any way. Masturbation is fun.
> —Dr. David Reuben

The reason I feel guilty about masturbation is that I'm so bad at it!
> —David Steinberg

I like to use the term "manipulation of the genitalia."
> —Police spokesman Bill Stookey
> on what Pee-wee Herman
> was caught doing in an adult
> theater

Men

The average man is more interested in a woman who is interested in him than he is in a woman with beautiful legs.
> —Marlene Dietrich

Beware of men who cry. It's true that men who cry are sensitive to and in touch with feelings, but the only feelings they tend to be sensitive to and in touch with are their own.
> —Nora Ephron

You never know a man until you know how he loves.
> —Sigmund Freud

Macho does not prove mucho.
> —Zsa Zsa Gabor

The only place men want depth in a woman is in her décolletage.

—Zsa Zsa Gabor

Women fail to understand how much men hate them.

—Germaine Greer

Men are those creatures with two legs and eight hands.

—Jayne Mansfield

There are two things no man will admit he can't do, drive and make love.

—Sterling Moss

Men are nicotine-soaked, beer-besmirched, whiskey-greased, red-eyed devils.

—Carry Nation

There is nothing more fun than a man.

—Dorothy Parker

I require three things in a man: he must be handsome, ruthless, and stupid.

—Dorothy Parker

You never know a guy until you've tried him in bed. You know more about a guy in one night in bed than you do in months of conversation. In the sack, they can't cheat.

—Edith Piaf

I find men terribly exciting and any girl who says she doesn't is an old maid, a streetwalker, or a saint.

—Lana Turner

It's not the men in my life that counts but the life in my men.
—Mae West

Give a man a free hand and he'll run it all over you.
—Mae West

A man I don't like doesn't exist.
—Mae West

I like two kinds of men: domestic and foreign.
—Mae West

Some men are all right in their place—if they only knew the right places.
—Mae West

Monogamy

For me, the highest level of sexual excitement is in a monogamous relationship.
—Warren Beatty

It destroys one's nerves to be amiable every day to the same human being.
—Benjamin Disraeli

God, for two people to be able to live together for the rest of their lives is almost unnatural.
—Jane Fonda

One who has mastered the art of monogamy.
> —Miss USA Shannon La Rhea
> on the type of man she wants
> to marry

Hard work is damn near as overrated as monogamy.
> —Huey P. Long

By nature, I am not monogamous. But I have been monogamous....I say monogamy doesn't make any difference; women suspect you whether it's true or not.
> —' ·k Nicholson

Monogamy: a synonym for monotony.
> —Gregory Nunn

I've only slept with men I've married. How many women can make that claim?
> —Elizabeth Taylor

By nature, I don't think man is monogamous, even though by agreement he tries to be.
> —John Travolta

Bigamy is having one husband too many. Monogamy is the same.
> —Oscar Wilde

Music

Rock and roll at its core is merely a bunch of raving shit.
> —Lester Baugs

The sound of a harpsichord—two skeletons copulating on a thin roof in a thunderstorm.

—Sir Thomas Beecham

I'm into pop because I want to get rich, get famous, and get laid.

—Bob Geldof

I know only two tunes, one of them is "Yankee Doodle," and the other one isn't.

—Ulysses S. Grant

Music played at weddings always reminds me of the music played for soldiers before they go into battle.

—Heinrich Heine

My music is supposed to make you wanna fuck.

—Janis Joplin

The opera is to music what a bawdy house is to a cathedral.

—H. L. Mencken

You ask any musician why he wants only to play jazz and he'll tell you the same thing.

—Dudley Moore on playing jazz to get women

I sing like shit.

—Rosie Perez on record companies offering her singing contracts

You can't take a fucking record like other people take the Bible.

—Keith Richards

To eat, to sing, to digest, and to love are four acts of the comic opera that is life.

—Gioacchino Rossini

Rock 'n' roll is the most brutal, ugly, vicious form of expression-sly, lewd, plain fact dirty...rancid smelling, aphrodisiac...the martial music of every delinquent on the face of the earth.

—Frank Sinatra

I think pop music has done more for oral intercourse than anything else that has ever happened, and vice versa.

—Frank Zappa

Nudity

It was the first time you got to see the actual star's organs. Big deal!

—Alan Bates on his nude
appearance in a movie

To be nude within the meaning of this ordinance means the absence of an opaque covering which covers the genitals, pubic hair, buttocks, perineum, anus, or anal region of any person or any portion of the breast at or below the areola thereof of any female person.

—Berkeley, California,
Ordinance No. 6199-N.S.,
effective August 19, 1993

I don't know. They were wearing a paper bag over their head.

—Yogi Berra when asked if a "streaker" was male or female

I have seen three emperors in their nakedness, and the sight was not inspiring.

—German Chancellor Otto von Bismarck

He's not going to come back nude. That's the bottom line.

—University of California on a student attending classes nude

For a woman to be loved, she usually ought to be naked.

—Pierre Cardin

If I don't have a tan, I feel naked.

—George Hamilton

Clearly there is more skin on TV than there was a few years ago.

—Walter Kendrick

I don't like dirty pictures. I'm glad nobody took their clothes off in our movies.

—Groucho Marx

Full frontal nudity...has now become accepted by every branch of the theatrical profession with the possible exception of lady accordian players.

—Denis Norden

I never expected to see the day when girls would get sunburned in the places they do today.
—Will Rogers

I think naked people are very nice. Posing nude is perhaps the best way of reaching people.
—Stella Stevens

My breasts aren't actresses.
—Liv Ullmann on nudity in the theater

A woman thinks she knows a man if she's seen him naked.
—Jimmy Williams

The sexiest thing in the world is to be totally naked with your wedding band on.
—Debra Winger

Nudity on the stage? I think it's disgusting, shameful, and unpatriotic. But if I were twenty-two with a great body, it would be artistic, tasteful, patriotic, and a progressive, religious experience.
—Shelley Winters

Observations and Opinions

If it's not erotic, it is not interesting.
—Fernando Arrabal

I wish I had invented sex. Sex is number one!
—Brigitte Bardot

Sex is not taxed—but it can be taxing.
—John Barrymore

The thing that takes up the least amount of time and causes the most amount of trouble is sex.
—John Barrymore

The sex life of a fish is nothing to brag about.
—Robert Benchley

Sex is like money—very nice to have but vulgar to talk about.
—Tonia Berg

To my mind, the two most fascinating subjects in the universe are sex and the eighteenth century.
—Brigid Brophy

If the world were a logical place, men would ride sidesaddle.
—Rita Mae Brown

It doesn't matter what you do in the bedroom as long as you don't do it in the street and frighten the horses.
—Mrs. Patrick Campbell

It was long accepted by the missionaries that morality was inversely proportional to the amount of clothing people wore.
—Alex Carey

The pleasure is momentary, the position ridiculous, and the expense damnable.
—Fourth Earl of Chesterfield

113

Sex ought to be wholly a satisfying link between two affectionate people from which they emerge unanxious, rewarded, and ready for more.

—Alex Comfort

Sex is no longer what men do to women and women are supposed to enjoy. Sexual interaction is a loving fusion.

—Alex Comfort

There are some things you can get in the mood for all the time and sex is one of them, if it's with the right person.

—Jimmy Connors

The act of sex, gratifying as it may be, is God's joke on humanity.

—Bette Davis

When people start sleeping with one another, it ruins things. Kaput!

—Marlene Dietrich

Sex is as important as food and drink.

—Britt Ekland

All mankind loves a lover.

—Ralph Waldo Emerson

There may be some things better than sex, and some things may be worse. But there is nothing exactly like it.

—W. C. Fields

Fish fuck in it.

—W. C. Fields on why he never
drank water

The more underdeveloped the country, the more overdeveloped the women.

—John Kenneth Galbraith

Sex will outlive us all.

—Sam Goldwyn

There are some things that are better than bad sex: peanut butter and jelly. But in general, I can't think of anything better than good sex.

—Billy Joel

The zipless fuck was more than a fuck... The zipless fuck is absolutely pure. It is free of ulterior motives. There is no power game. The man is not "taking" and the woman is not "giving." No one is attempting to cuckold a husband or humiliate a wife. No one is trying to prove anything or get anything out of anyone. The zipless fuck is the purest thing there is. And it is rarer than the unicorn.

—Erica Jong

Sex is good, but not as good as fresh sweet corn.

—Garrison Keillor

I find the three major administrative problems on a campus are sex for the students, athletics for the alumni, and parking for the faculty.

—School administrator Clark Kerr

Whatever else can be said about sex, it cannot be called a dignified performance.

—Helen Lawrenson

It is nothing less than astonishing to discover how many women [and] well-informed couples still believe the Victorian idea that there is something called the "sex act" and that a man does it to a woman.

—Masters and Johnson

My own belief is that there is hardly anyone whose sexual life, if it were broadcast, would not fill the world at large with surprise and horror.

—W. Somerset Maugham

Fucky-wucky! It's not the simple pastime it would seem to be.

—Henry Miller

Hollywood's a place where they'll pay you a thousand dollars for a kiss and fifty cents for your soul.

—Marilyn Monroe

I think sex is the most important part of anybody's life.

—Dudley Moore

Sex—the poor man's polo.

—Clifford Odets

I'm very much in touch with my feminine side...Women don't always want to be manhandled. A lot of times they want to be made love to by a man who can do it softly, like a woman.

—Luke Perry

There is no greater nor keener pleasure than that of bodily love—and none which is more irrational.

—Plato

Love is two minutes fifty-two seconds of squishing noises.
It shows your mind isn't clicking right.
—Johnny Rotten

Unless she's bright, once you go to bed with her, there's
nothing to talk about.
—Peter Sellers

The world's books get written, its pictures printed, its
statues modeled, its symphonies composed, by people
who are free from the otherwise universal dominion of the
tyranny of sex.
—George Bernard Shaw

The word "screw" conjures up a mind-boggling image. The
man on top, revolving horizontally in a continuous spiral
motion, with one Frankensteinian objective—to
permanently attach the lady to the bed.
—Alan Sherman

There are only two superlative compliments you can
receive from a woman. "I think you're a master chef" and
"I think you're a great lay." The two basic drives in life.
—Rod Steiger

Sex, treated properly, can be one of the most gorgeous
things in the world.
—Elizabeth Taylor

Is it possible that blondes also prefer gentlemen?
—Mamie Van Doren

Sex is. There is nothing more to be done about it. Sex builds no roads, writes no novels, and sex certainly gives no meaning to anything in life but itself.

—Gore Vidal

Sex is the biggest nothing of all time.

—Andy Warhol

There is no difference.

—Andy Warhol on the difference between art and eroticism

Healthy, lusty sex is wonderful.

—John Wayne

We made civilization in order to impress our girlfriends.

—Orson Welles

Sex is an emotion in motion.

—Mae West

When women go wrong, men go right after them.

—Mae West

Women fuck to love and men love to fuck.

—Jimmy Williams

On Others, Compliments

He was as much a perfectionist in his lovemaking as he was in his juggling. He never dropped a cigar box accidentally, and by the same token, he never fumbled during a golden moment.

—Mistress of W. C. Fields

Sleeping with Kurt Cobain is worth a half million dollars.

—Courtney Love, widow of rock group Nirvana leader

I'd like to do a love scene with him just to see what all the yelling is about.

—Shirley MacLaine on her brother Warren Beatty

If someone tells Kemp he's a bad motherfucker, he knows that's a compliment.

—John McKay on Jack Kemp

He is the least weird man I've ever known.

—Elizabeth Taylor on Michael Jackson

On Others, Insults

I said that I didn't think Chevy Chase could ad-lib a fart after a baked bean dinner. I think he took umbrage at that a little bit.

—Johhny Carson

My, that's got every fire hydrant in America worried.
—Bill Clinton on Dan Quayle's
intentions of being the "pit
bull" in helping elect George
Bush in 1992

I babysit his girlfriends.
—Jamie Lee Curtis on her father
Tony

When I want to play with a prick, I'll play with my own.
—W. C. Fields on why he
refused to play golf with a
film bigshot

A plumber's idea of Cleopatra.
—W. C. Fields on Mae West

They don't have a page that broad.
—Gennifer Flowers on why
Hillary Clinton could not pose
nude in *Penthouse*

Hubert Humphrey talks so fast that listening to him is like
trying to read *Playboy* magazine with your wife turning
the pages.
—Barry Goldwater

Where I come from, we have Cuomo the homo and then in
New York City, Dinkins the pinkins.
—Peter Grace on why he moved
his company from New York

LBJ always referred to Robert Kennedy in one way. He called him "the little shit." I'll buy that in spades although in that connection I wouldn't have called him "little."
—Jimmy Hoffa

Jerry Ford is a nice guy, but he played too much football with his helmet off.
—Lyndon B. Johnson

I'd rather have him inside the tent pissing out, than outside pissing in.
—Lyndon B. Johnson on J. Edgar Hoover

[Dick] Cavett has a much bigger cock and is a better lay than [Joe] Namath.
—Janis Joplin

Those guys from Kiss couldn't wipe their ass by themselves.
—Alan Lanier on rock group Kiss

...a pig, an ass, a dunghill, a lying buffoon, a mad fool with a frothy mouth, a blubbery ass, a fanatic, madman....
—Martin Luther on Henry VIII

Joe has great respect for girls. Only last week in New York, he saved a girl from being attacked. He controlled himself.
—Dean Martin on Joe Namath

A pipsqueak who didn't have the talent of a butterfly's fart.

—Walter Matthau on Barbra
Streisand

He sure likes to touch his peeper a lot, doesn't he? I think he looks like a girl.

—Eight-year-old Erik Nelson on
Michael Jackson's "Black on
White" video

That fucking bastard, he wasn't supposed to use notes.

—Richard M. Nixon on JFK and
the TV debates

That asshole.

—Richard M. Nixon on
Canadian Prime Minister
Pierre Trudeau

Poor George [Bush], he can't help it—he was born with a silver foot in his mouth.

—Ann Richards, governor of
Texas

Jackie Onassis, with her eyes on either side of her head like E.T., is not fair game? With her 38 million dollars?
—Joan Rivers

I know Don Johnson and he is scum. He's just a long-haired guy with good looks who makes a bundle selling sex, drugs, and violence on commercial television.
—Jay Rockefeller

It's a great book, but I wouldn't want to shake hands with the author.

> —Jacqueline Susann on the novel *Portnoy's Complaint*

Nixon is a shifty-eyed goddam liar, and people know it. He's one of the few in the history of this country to run for high office talking out of both sides of his mouth at the same time and lying out of both sides.

> —Harry S. Truman

Do you mind if I sit back a little? Because your breath is very bad.

> —Donald Trump to Larry King on CNN

First in war, first in peace, first in the pants of his countrywomen.

> —Woodrow Wilson on George Washington

God would have been merciful if He had given him a little teeny penis so that he could get on with his life.

> —Sean Young on actor James Woods

On Themselves

I don't think anyone conceives of sex the way I do: surrealistic and rich with humor.

> —Woody Allen

I have been one of the great lovers of my century.

> —Sarah Bernhardt

Maybe I'm not talented...the square people think I'm too hip and the hip people think I'm too square. And nobody likes my choice of men—everybody thinks I'm fucking the Mormon Tabernacle Choir.

—Cher

I'm a very masculine person even if some people have their doubts.

—Boy George

I've always looked better lying down.

—Jerry Hall

There was a time in my life when I spent 90 percent of my money on booze and broads. And the rest of it I just wasted.

—Ben Jones

I have a face like the behind of an elephant.

—Charles Laughton

I'm a bit of a prude myself.

—Gypsy Rose Lee

I've made so many movies playing a hooker that they don't pay me in the regular way anymore. They leave it on the dresser.

—Shirley MacLaine

I'm interested in pushing people's buttons.

—Madonna on her down-and-dirty style

Power is a great aphrodisiac and I'm a very powerful person.

—Madonna

I'm as confident as Cleopatra's pussy.

—Bette Midler

Anyone who is against me will look like a rat, unless I run off with Eddie Fisher.

—Jackie Kennedy (Onassis)

I've got sagging breasts and a low-slung ass...but I can still get men.

—Edith Piaf

I love tap dancing because you can stamp your little guts out if you're pissed off.

—Gilda Radner

I am not a ball-busting, castrating bitch.

—Roseanne

I like sexual intercourse because of its amazing power of producing a celestial flood of emotion and exaltation of existence which, however momentary, gave me a sample of what may one day be the normal state of being for mankind in intellectual ecstasy.

—George Bernard Shaw

I never miss a chance to have sex or appear on television.

—Gore Vidal

It isn't what I do but how I do it. It isn't what I say but how I say it. And how I look when I do it.

—Mae West

I do all my best work in bed.
>—Mae West

I've known so many men, the FBI ought to come to me for fingerprints.
>—Mae West

When I'm good, I'm very good; when I'm bad, I'm better.
>—Mae West

I have only done what comes naturally, what the average American does secretly, drenching himself in guilt fixations and phobias because of his sense of sinning. I have never committed what I would call sin.
>—Mae West

All the things I like to do are either immoral, illegal, or fattening.
>—Alexander Woollcott

Oral Sex

My wife gives good headache.
>—Rodney Dangerfield

Not every woman can deep-throat a man. But don't worry. Just concentrate on the upper half of a man's penis, while you're fondling the other part with your hands.
>—Xaviera Hollander

I regret to say that we are powerless to act in cases of oral-genital intimacy, unless it has obstructed interstate commerce.
>—J. Edgar Hoover

Many women have the gut feeling that their genitals are ugly. One reason women are gratified by oral-genital relations is that it's a way of a man saying "I like your cunt. I can eat it."

—Erica Jong

You know why most men lose their hair? That's what comes from fighting your way under tight nightgowns.

—Beatrice Lillie

Deep Throat was really just me, acting naturally.

—Linda Lovelace

Older guys like to receive head, but they don't like to give it.

—Victoria Principal

I rowed us to a secluded spot.... Right there, the estranged First Lady of Canada lent new meaning to the term "head of state."

—Geraldo Rivera on his alleged
affair with Margaret Trudeau

Never do with your hands what you could do better with your mouth.

—Rock groupie Cherrie Vanilla

If your cock's as big as your mouth, honey, I'll see you after the show.

—Mae West to a heckler

I don't care for active oral sex. I do it to accommodate the other person. But if the other person has a large member, I choke. I can't do more than five minutes of it.
—Tennessee Williams

Orgasms

At the moment of climax, there is a oneness with you and your husband and with God....When you come together, it's like when the church is brought up to meet Christ in the air.
—Anita Bryant

Like the tickling feeling you get inside your nose before you sneeze.
—Children's sex manual on the orgasm

Like a slight attack of apoplexy.
—Democritus on the orgasm

He regarded every orgasm as his testimony of love for me.
—Britt Ekland on Rod Stewart

Is there a way to accept the concept of the female orgasm and still command the respect of your foreign auto mechanic?
—Bruce Feinstein

In the case of some women, orgasms take quite a bit of time. Before signing on with such a partner, make sure you are willing to lay aside, say, the month of June, with sandwiches having to be brought in.
—Bruce Jay Friedman

One thinks of college girls working out their orgasm averages.

—Anthony Glyn on how the
British view American girls

[I saw] in the human sperm, two naked thighs, the legs, the breast, both arms, etc.

—Stephen Hamm on what he
saw in his microscope

The number of available orgasms is fixed at birth and can be expended. A man should make love very seldom, or he will have nothing left for middle age.

—Ernest Hemingway

Basically, a man's and a woman's orgasms are similar, consisting of an immensely pleasurable series of muscular contractions, succeeded by a feeling of total relaxation.

—Xaviera Hollander

Laughter is an orgasm triggered by the intercourse of reason and unreason.

—Jack Kroll

And you've spent enough in me to float one.

—Lillie Langtry responding to
the Prince of Wales's comment
"I've spent enough on you to
buy a battleship."

If I like what the actor is doing to me, I don't have any trouble coming while the camera is rolling.

—Hyapatia Lee

If you don't have an orgasm daily, you become very nervous, very uptight. I do, anyway.

—Linda Lovelace

There can be back of the neck orgasms, bottom of the foot orgasms, and palm of the hand orgasms.

—Masters and Johnson

A man must be potent and orgasmic to ensure the future of the race. A woman only needs to be available.

—Masters and Johnson

Making love, we are all more alike than we are talking or acting. In the climax of the sexual act, moreover, we forget ourselves. That is commonly felt to be one of its recommendations. Sex annihilates identity.

—Mary McCarthy

An orgasm has replaced the cross as the focus of longing and the image of fulfillment.

—Malcolm Muggeridge

A great portion [of semen] comes from the brain.

—Ambrose Pare (1513)

You can, after all, produce an orgasm yourself if that's what you want, so we must go to bed for something more.

—Merle Shain

A show is like having an orgasm. It's like having an incredible, natural climax. And then suddenly, it's all finished, and you don't know what to do next.

—Rod Stewart

An orgasm is just a reflex like a sneeze.
—Dr. Ruth Westheimer

Orgies

I believe that sex is a beautiful thing between two people. Between five, it's fantastic.
—Woody Allen

A famous guy came up to me. He had his arms around two girls and he invited me to join the threesome at his house, where we'd all get into his hot tub. He said his hot tub was so full of sperm, you could practically walk on it! That was supposed to turn me on! Plus the fact that it would have been an orgy.
—Morgan Fairchild

Home is heaven and orgies are vile. But you need an orgy once in a while.
—Ogden Nash

You get a better class of person at orgies, because people have to keep in trim more. There is an awful lot of going around holding in your stomach, you know. Everybody is polite to each other. The conversation isn't very good but you can't have everything.
—Gore Vidal

Penis Envy

No woman ever went through penis envy. We never did. The books say we're supposed to but look who wrote the books. We never had penis envy. But men have womb envy, because we are directly connected to life and we give life.

—Yoko Ono

Philosophies

The duration of passion is proportional with the original resistance of the woman.

—Honoré de Balzac

Every time you think you got it made, old Mother Nature kicks you in the scrotum.

—Robert Blake

The ability to make love frivolously is the chief characteristic which distinguishes human beings from beasts.

—Heywood Broun

I ejaculate, therefore I am.

—Quentin Crisp

Always look out for number one and be careful not to step in number two.

—Rodney Dangerfield

The act of procreation and the members employed therein are so repulsive that if it were not for the beauty of the faces...the adornments...the pent-up impulse, nature would lose the human species.

—Leonardo da Vinci

Sex is as important as a cheese sandwich. But a cheese sandwich, if you ain't got one in your belly, is extremely important.

—Ian Drury

Much of our highly valued cultured heritage has been acquired at the cost of sexuality.

—Sigmund Freud

If you fuck a bull, you get bullshit on your prick.

—Paul Goodman

Anything that can't be done in bed isn't worth doing at all.

—Joey Heatherton

While you're saving your face, you're losing your ass.

—Lyndon B. Johnson

Power is the ultimate aphrodisiac.

—Henry Kissinger

The future will see sex become the unifying art form, the basic vocation/avocation, the harmonious combination of our intellectual, sensual, neurological, genital potentialities.

—Timothy Leary

Sex is the metaphor that I use, but for me, it's about love. It's about tolerance, acceptance and saying, "Look, everybody has different needs and wants and preferences and desires and fantasies. And we should not damn somebody or judge somebody because it's different than yours."

—Madonna

Philosophy is to the real world as masturbation is to sex.

—Karl Marx

The higher you climb the flagpole, the more people see your rear end.

—Don Meredith

I wanted to say something about the universe. There's God, angels, planets...and horseshit.

—Zero Mostel

If you aren't going all the way, why go at all?

—Joe Namath

So many people go through life without a direction. They go from stop to stop. It's like they're on a bus and the only time they get off is to piss.

—Todd Rundgren

Life is a shit sandwich and every day you take another bite.

—Joe Schmidt

If a man can fuck and drive race cars, man, I mean, what else is there?

—Billy Scott

Familiarity breeds contempt—and children.
>—Mark Twain

Whenever I'm caught between two evils, I take the one I've never tried.
>—Mae West

To err is human—but it feels divine.
>—Mae West

Life is a shit sandwich. But, man, if you've got enough bread, you don't taste the shit.
>—Jonathan Winters

Politics

I can conceive of nothing worse than a man-governed world—except a woman-governed world.
>—Lady Nancy Astor

Fuck them. They didn't vote for us.
>—James Baker, former
>Secretary of State on Jewish
>critics

If presidents don't do it to their wives, they do it to the country.
>—Mel Brooks

I don't want to be charged with child abuse.
>—Pat Buchanan on why he
>avoided an argument with
>Dan Quayle

If this doesn't work, I'm going to be the pissedest-off guy around.

—George Bush on his efforts to
land the VP spot on the 1980
GOP ticket

I think the American people want a solemn ass as President. And I think I'll go along with them.

—Calvin Coolidge

We are finally going to wrassle to the ground this giant orgasm that is just out of control.

—Senator Dennis DeConcini on
a constitutional amendment to
balance the federal budget

Nothing short of being caught in bed with a dead girl or a live boy can hurt my political career in this state.

—Governor of Louisiana Edwin
C. Edwards

The Vice President ain't worth a pitcher of warm piss.

—John Nance Gardner, VP
under FDR

If everybody in this town connected with politics had to leave town because of [chasing women] and drinking, you'd have no government.

—Barry Goldwater

The Christine Jorgensen of politics.

—Senator Charles Goodell on
Vice President Spiro Agnew

The appointment of a woman to office is an innovation for which the public is not prepared, nor am I.
—Thomas Jefferson

Boys, I may not know much, but I know the difference between chicken shit and chicken salad.
—Lyndon B. Johnson

I never trust a man until I've got his pecker in my pocket.
—Lyndon B. Johnson

Jerry Ford can't fart and chew gum at the same time.
—Lyndon B. Johnson

The Democrats are doing it to their secretaries and the Republicans are doing it to the country.
—Joan Mondale

As long as I am in the White House, there will be no relaxation of the national effort to control and eliminate smut from our national life.
—Richard Nixon

Those who are too smart to engage in politics are punished by being governed by those who are dumber.
—Plato

The legitimate job [of Washington] is always second to the blow job.
—Liz Ray

Politics is supposed to be the second oldest profession, but I have an idea it has become the first.
—Ronald Reagan

It is about a socialist, anti-family political movement that encourages women to leave their husbands, kill their children, practice witchcraft, destroy capitalism, and become lesbians.

—Pat Robertson on the ERA
amendment

I think it's about time we voted for senators with breasts. After all, we've been voting for boobs long enough.

—Arizona senatorial candidate
Claire Sargent

People would say we need a man on the ticket.

—Pat Schroeder on why Bush
would not choose a woman
for a running mate in 1988

Don't vote for that fucking Bush!

—Bruce Springsteen

I never gave them hell, I just tell the truth and they think it's hell.

—Harry S. Truman

Reader, suppose you were an idiot; and suppose you were a member of Congress, but I repeat myself.

—Mark Twain

There's a huge push of bimbo fever.

—Betsy Wright on Democratic
efforts to defuse rumors of
Bill Clinton's extramarital
affairs

They seemed to be saying, "Here, I've got breasts. Vote for me!"

—Larry Yatch on 1992 female candidates

Pornography

Pornography...is presumably intended to arouse sexual desire and procure solitary orgasm, against which, so far as I know, there has never been any law except that of a scout master.

—Anthony Burgess

I think it quite likely that there is no such thing as good pornography. If it's good, then it's not pornography.

—Vincent Canby

I don't think pornography is very harmful, but it is terribly, terribly boring.

—Noël Coward

I would like to suggest that, at least on the face of it, a stroke-by-stroke story of copulation is exactly as absurd as a chew-by-chew account of the consumption of a chicken wing.

—William Gass

In the consumer limbo of adult entertainment, a clever title or an alluring photo on the front of the video package is all you need to sell the tape.

—Al Goldstein

If porno is your bag, you don't have much imagination of your own.

—Sol Gordon

That's not photography—that's pornography.
—Hugh Hefner on the first appearance of pubic hair in *Penthouse* magazine

My reaction to porno films is as follows: After the first ten minutes, I want to go home and screw. After the first twenty minutes, I never want to screw again as long as I live.

—Erica Jong

What is pornography to one man is the laughter of genius to another.

—D. H. Lawrence

The difference between pornography and erotica is lighting.

—Gloria Leonard

When the movies started delivering messages, they lost their charisma. Now the messages are being replaced by porno. Between the two, porno is better.

—Anita Loos

It makes me so mad that sex films are called obscene when movies full of slaughter are rated PG. Kids learn that killing is accepted; what they should learn is that sex is good.

—Linda Lovelace

If the purpose of pornography is to excite sexual desire, it is unnecessary for the young, inconvenient for the middle-aged, and unseemly for the old.
—Malcolm Muggeridge

Americans don't like sex movies, they like sexy movies.
—Jack Nicholson

At last, an unprintable book that is fit to be read.
—Ezra Pound on *Tropic of Cancer*

I don't believe the Founding Fathers ever intended to create a nation where the rights of pornographers would take precedence over the rights of parents.
—Ronald Reagan

I want to be the Shirley MacLaine of porno.
—Annie Sprinkle

I know it when I see it.
—Supreme Court Justice Potter Stewart on pornography

Western man, especially the Western critic, still finds it very hard to go into print and say, "I recommend you go and see this because it gave me an erection."
—Kenneth Tynan

We wanted to be the Walt Disney of porn.
—Andy Warhol

Pornography, art, and entertainment presented with all the charm of open brain surgery.

—Jimmy Williams

Pregnancy

Being pregnant is a very boring six months. I am not particularly maternal. It's an occupational hazard of being a wife.

—Princess Anne

I wish I could say it was immaculate conception, but it wasn't.

—Lynn Delano on two South Dakota prisoners who became pregnant

It is now possible for a flight attendant to get a pilot pregnant.

—Richard J. Ferris

I've got more paternity suits than leisure suits.

—Engelbert Humperdinck

This is not an ordinary pregnancy.

—Antonio Periquet on a hermaphrodite who, legally a male, was about to have a baby

I called the doctor, and he told me that the contraptions were an hour apart.

—Mackey Sasser on his wife's progress in labor

It is true that when I was fourteen years old I became pregnant. The baby was born prematurely and died shortly after the birth. The experience was the most emotional, confusing, and traumatic of my young life.

—Oprah Winfrey

Premenstrual Syndrome (PMS)

Now we've got all these men out there worrying that we'll all have PMS on the same day and blow up the town.

—Barbara Carr on the four new councilwomen in Pacifica, California

You can't accept one individual's [criticism], particularly if it's a female. When they get their period it's difficult for them to function as normal human beings.

—Jerry Lewis on a bad review

Women complain about premenstrual syndrome, but I think of it as the only time of the month I can be myself.

—Roseanne

If women are supposed to be less rational and more emotional at the beginning of our menstrual cycle when their female hormone is at its lowest level, then why isn't it logical to say that in those few days, women behave the most like the way men behave all month long?

—Gloria Steinem

143

Men may have wars, but women have their period.
                                        —Robin Williams

Press

Ask about our cup size or favorite position, but please—
no personal questions.

>   —Shane Barbi, who appeared
>   on the cover of *Playboy* with
>   her twin sister, when the press
>   asked who was older

The only time I worry is when I'm fishing. When I'm
standing in the river for hours, I sometimes have a pee in
the water. And I'm always petrified some cameraman is
going to catch me at it.

                                        —Prince Charles

According to the press, I was Lady Bountiful of the sheets.
                                        —Doris Day

Don't tell the bastards anything.

>   —William Faulkner when his
>   agent asked for a
>   biographical sketch for the
>   press

They've asked me everything but how I sleep with my
husband. And if they asked me that, I would have told
them, as often as possible.

                                        —First Lady Betty Ford

144

Jack Anderson is the lowest form of human being to walk the earth. He's a muckraker who lies, steals, and let me tell you this, Mr. [John] Dean, he'll go lower than dog shit for a story.

—J. Edgar Hoover

Katie Graham is going to get her teat caught in a big fat wringer.

—John Mitchell on the
Washington Post's pursual of
the Watergate story

When they use a proctoscope, it's going too far.

—Richard M. Nixon on media
scrutiny

Well, did you do any fornicating this weekend?

—Richard M. Nixon to David
Frost before an interview

I wish I had as much in bed as I get in the newspapers.

—Linda Ronstadt

I don't talk to you white motherfuckers...you bitch motherfuckers in the white press....Fuck you, you motherfucking assholes.

—Gus Savage to a white
reporter

Profanity

Bullshit!

—Mel Brooks on the accusation
that he's vulgar

Deep doo-doo.
>—George Bush on bad trouble

We just screwed all these people.
>—Hillary Rodham Clinton to
>husband Bill at a White House
>open house

All pro athletes are bilingual. They speak English and profanity.
>—Gordie Howe

We are not taught to think decently on sex objects, and consequently we have no language for them except indecent language.
>—George Bernard Shaw

Under certain circumstances, profanity provides a relief denied even to prayer.
>—Mark Twain

Professions/Careers

I'm not the first straight dancer or the last.
>—Mikhail Baryshnikov

The only people with a right to complain about what I do for a living are vegetarian nudists.
>—Fur trapper Ken Bates

I love playing bitches.
>—Joan Crawford

I'm plenty proud of Hollywood....I'd say if you want to grow a plant, put it where there's some good horseshit around to grow it in.
—Kirk Douglas

In the sex field, you can be totally stupid and still make money.
—Al Goldstein

I would rather score a touchdown than make love to the prettiest girl in the United States.
—Paul Hornung

The work was arduous and humiliating.
—Lauren Hutton on working as a Playboy bunny

I'd rather hit than have sex.
—Reggie Jackson

There is nothing like actually getting on stage. It's the biggest buzz of all for me. It's like fucking for two hours.
—Elton John

I've spread my legs in the back seat in a creative sense quite a few times.
—Stephen King

No one ever got to be a star by fucking somebody. It just doesn't happen.
—Donna Mills

A game is a closed field, a ring of death with, uh, sex at the center. Performing is the only game I've got.
—Jim Morrison

I love football, it's the second best thing in the world
—Joe Namath

I could have made a fortune as a dominatrix.
—Camille Paglia

I never made any money until I took my pants off.
—Sally Rand

Don't get married to an actress, because they're also actresses in bed.
—Roberto Rossellini

My choice early in life was either to be a piano player in a whorehouse or a politician. And to tell the truth, there's hardly a difference.
—Harry S. Truman

I didn't get ahead by sleeping with people. Girls, take heart!
—Barbara Walters

I adore football players; their passes are so forward.
—Mae West

When I act I don't make love and when I make love I don't act.
—Mae West

Because it usually means you're either fucking or working—and what else is there?
—Debra Winger

Boy meets girl, girl gets boy into a pickle, boy gets pickle into girl.

— Jack Woodford on how to plot
a story

I don't play lesbians, honey. Not this kid.
— Jane Wyman on acceptable
roles

Promiscuity

The sad lesson of life is that you treat a girl like that with respect, and the next guy comes along and he's banging the hell out of her.

— Art Buchwald

The chief occupation of my life has been to cultivate the pleasures of the senses. Feeling myself born for the fair sex, I have always loved it, and have been loved in return as often as possible.

— Casanova

Yes, that's correct—20,000 different ladies. At my age that equals out to having sex with 1.2 women a day, every day since I was fifteen.

— Wilt Chamberlain

It's hard to take showers with only one of the five guys you're dating.

— Cher

Hell, if I'd jumped all the dames I'm supposed to have jumped, I'd never have had time to go fishing.

— Clark Gable

I think any man in business would be foolish to fool around with his secretary. If it's somebody else's secretary, fine.

—Barry Goldwater

It's a good thing I wasn't born a girl, because I never could say no.

—Warren G. Harding

They have gone from puritanism into promiscuity without passing through sensuality.

—Molly Haskell

Just because a man has something that sticks out doesn't mean he's got to put it anywhere and everywhere.

—Goldie Hawn

I'm saving the bass player for Omaha.

—Janis Joplin on a long train ride

Who's Virginia?

—Rose Kennedy when told her daughter-in-law Joan lived in Boston and her son Ted lived in Virginia

What is a promiscuous person? It's usually someone who is getting more sex than you are.

—Victor Lownes

I've always found promiscuous women interesting. I suspect I would have been promiscuous if I'd been a woman. I certainly have been as a man.

—Norman Mailer

I have a wife and a mistress. From my wife I get love and understanding and sensitivity. From my mistress I get love and passion and sensuality.
—Marcello Mastroianni

Women of my generation, unlike generations before us, we have been with several men—or in some cases, many men. I raise the question, why?
—Joni Mitchell

I did not sleep. I never do when I am over-happy, over-unhappy, or in bed with a strange man.
—Edna O'Brien

I want a person who's in a senior position busy serving the people, not chasing around at night, trying to toe-dance between his responsibilities to his family and his latest hot chick.
—H. Ross Perot on hiring promiscuous people

Personally, I like sex and I don't care what a man thinks of me as long as I get what I want from him—which is usually sex.
—Valerie Perrine

My schoolmates would make love to anything that moved, but I never saw any reason to limit myself.
—Emo Philips

A man can sleep around, no questions asked. But if a woman makes nineteen or twenty mistakes, she's a tramp.
—Joan Rivers

All right, ladies, any girl who doesn't want to fuck can leave right now.

—Babe Ruth entering a party

If I had as many love affairs as you have given me credit for, I would now be speaking to you from a jar in the Harvard Medical School.

—Frank Sinatra

It ain't sex that's troublesome, it's staying up all night looking for it.

—Casey Stengel

I can understand companionship. I can understand bought sex in the afternoon. I cannot understand the love affair.

—Gore Vidal

I've been on more laps than a napkin.

—Mae West

Fifty men outside? I'm tired. Send ten of them home.

—Mae West

Prostitution

The women who take husbands not out of love but out of greed, to get their bills paid, to get a fine house and clothes and jewels; the women who marry to get out of a tiresome job, or to get away from disagreeable relatives, or to avoid being called an old maid—these are whores in everything but name. The only difference between them and my girls is that my girls gave a man his money's worth.

—Polly Adler

I was naughty, I wasn't bad. Bad is hurting people. Naughty is being amusing.

—Sydney Biddle Barrows

Prostitutes are necessary. Without them, men would assault respectable women on the streets.

—Napoleon Bonaparte

I would like to be a beautiful male prostitute.

—Lord Byron

A millionaire falling in love with a beautiful prostitute— what better story can they have than that?

—Charlie Chaplin

Sex is the great amateur art. The professional, male or female, is frowned upon. He or she misses the whole point and spoils the show.

—David Cort

The big difference between sex for money and sex for fun is that sex for money usually costs less.

—Brendan Francis

You can no longer just put prostitutes on. It has to be prostitutes who are sex addicts.

—Ed Glaven, a producer for
Donahue

I believe that sex is the most beautiful, natural, and wholesome thing that money can buy.
—Steve Martin

You can lead a horticulture but you can't make her think.
—Dorothy Parker

I can't take dictation. I can't type. I can't even answer the phone.
—Liz Ray, whose only responsibility as a government-paid employee of Congressman Wayne Hays was to sexually satisfy him

Many a marriage hardly differs from prostitution, except being harder to escape from.
—Bertrand Russell

Gimme four steaks, a dozen eggs, pound of bacon, three kegs of beer, fifteen potatoes, eighteen whores, seven cigars, and a dish of chocolate ice cream.
—Babe Ruth ordering dinner

Romance without finance is a nuisance. Few men value free merchandise. Let the chippies fall where they may.
—Sally Stanford

Prostitution, like acting, is being ruined by amateurs.
—Alexander Woollcott

Race

A black man should be killed if he's messing with a white woman.

—Muhammad Ali

First, a tight pussy, second, loose shoes, and third, a warm place to shit.

—Earl Butz on what blacks want. The comments cost Butz his job as secretary of agriculture

It's tough to find a secure black man who doesn't feel threatened that your career might serve to deball him.

—Diahann Carroll

There ain't nothin' in the whole world worse than an ugly white woman.

—Redd Foxx

Something is dismally wrong with an America in which a white prostitute can buy a house where a black man can't.

—Reverend Theodore Hesburgh

I know exactly what it feels like to get instantly horny for a black man.

—Xaviera Hollander

If you haven't had a chocolate-covered dwarf in your shower, you haven't lived.

—Kathy Self, former girlfriend of Herve Villechaize, who starred of *Fantasy Island*

I loved talking with my black friends about sex. They'd go into vivid descriptions without any shame at all. I loved it because it satisfied my voyeurism.

—John Travolta

Rape

Rape is nothing more or less than a conscious process of intimidation by which all men keep all women in a state of fear.

—Susan Brownmiller

I say this a lot, and I probably shouldn't; the difference between rape and seduction is salesmanship.

—Bill Carpenter

Damn it, when you get married, you kind of expect you're going to get a little sex.

—Jeremiah Denton on the prosecution of a man accused of raping his wife

Date rape, I assure you, lies in our medium-term future.

—P. Jay Fetner on why women should not be allowed in Yale's "Skull and Bones" club

All men are rapists and that's all they are. They rape us with their eyes, their laws, and their codes.

—Marilyn French

I think when a person has been found guilty of rape he should be castrated. That would stop him pretty quick.

—Billy Graham

The boys never meant any harm against the girls. They just meant to rape.

—Joyce Kithira, deputy
principal of the Kenyan
boarding school where
seventy-one girls were raped
and nineteen killed

That woman that is suing him is a bitch. I don't care if he raped her. He should learn about himself and why he behaves like that. But equally, she should look at herself and look at the disgrace she is making of women.

—Sinead O'Connor on Desiree
Washington, who was raped
by Mike Tyson

She never told me to stop, she never said I was hurting her, she never said no, nothing.

—Mike Tyson about his rape
victim

She told me to wear a condom, so I did. We were making love after that.

—Joel Valdez on his defense of
rape charges

I'm saying, "Listen, stop. That's not what I want." He was really forceful....It was just a battle that, I'm sorry to say, I lost. It was absolutely against my will and it was all over in two minutes.

—Schene Walters, former movie
starlet on an encounter with
Ronald Reagan in 1951

If it's inevitable, just relax and enjoy it.

> —Texas gubernatorial
> candidate Clayton Williams
> on rape

Relativity

When a man sits with a pretty girl for an hour, it seems like a minute. But let him sit on a hot stove for a minute—and it's longer than any hour. That's relativity.

> —Albert Einstein

Religion

God created women only to tame men.

> —Brigitte Bardot

I like convents, but I wish they wouldn't take any woman under the age of fifty.

> —Napoleon Bonaparte

Jewish women don't fuck back.

> —Mel Brooks

My lesbianism is an act of Christian charity. All those women out there are praying for a man, and I'm giving them my share.

> —Rita Mae Brown

If you believe there is a God, a God that made your body, and yet you think you can do anything with that body that's dirty, then the fault lies with the manufacturer.

> —Lenny Bruce

I have a great respect for someone from a strict Catholic upbringing who can climax without reservation.
—Robert Downey Jr.

How did sex come to be thought of as dirty in the first place? God must have been a Republican.
—Will Durst

It's just as Christian to get down on your knees for sex as it is for religion.
—Larry Flynt

If there is a God, I'm sure He's jerking off to *Screw*.
—Al Goldstein, editor of *Screw* magazine

Pray, good people, be civil; I am the Protestant whore.
—Nell Gwynn, mistress of Charles II, to an angry crowd in 1675

I think the essense of Judaio/Christian teachings is very similar to *Playboy.*
—Hugh Hefner

Woody Allen was right when someone asked him if he thought sex was dirty and he said, "If you do it right." Sex is not some sort of pristine, reverent ritual. You want reverent and pristine, go to church.
—Cynthia Heimel

The good news is that Jesus is coming back. The bad news is that He's really pissed off.
—Bob Hope

What can you say about a society that says God is dead and Elvis is alive?

—Irv Kupcinet

'Tis the devil inspires this evanescent ardor, in order to divert the parties from prayer.

—Martin Luther

Sex is one of the nine reasons for reincarnation...the other eight are unimportant.

—Henry Miller

Why should we take advice on sex from the Pope? If he knows anything about it, he shouldn't.

—George Bernard Shaw

Safe Sex

There's no such thing as safe sex. I really believe that. There may be semi-safe sex, but I don't think you can really say it's safe.

—Barbara Bush

We practice safe sex. We gave up the chandelier a long time ago.

—Kathy Lee Gifford on sex with her husband

Do not have sex with people you do not know and whose state you cannot attest to.

—Former Surgeon General C. Everett Koop

Make war, not love. It's safer.
—Henny Youngman

Seduction

Maybe if I hadn't been so fastidious, I might have changed history. But, oh, that body odor of his.
—Lina Basquette on Adolf
Hitler's attempt to seduce her

Love doesn't drop on you unexpectedly, you have to give off signals, sort of like an amateur radio operator.
—Helen Gurley Brown

He spread my legs and slid his cock up and into me. His hips moved smoothly and steadily, in and out...for the first time in my life, fucking a man felt good to me.
—Mrs. Lenny Bruce on her
husband

I was signing books and a very nice looking lady came by and said, "Mr. President, if you're still lusting in your heart, I'm available." The whole crowd broke out in laughter. I blushed.
—Jimmy Carter

Lovemaking is a sublime art that needs practice if it's to be true and significant. But I suspect you're going to be an excellent student.
—Charlie Chaplin on
deflowering his bride-to-be

I haven't met him but I send him naked pictures.
—Sheena Easton on her crush
on Peter Jennings

She was the sophisticated older woman and I was the inexperienced boy, just like in one of her movies.
—Eddie Fisher on his affair with
Marlene Dietrich

She who is silent consents.
—French proverb

I tried to charm the pants off Bob Dylan but everyone will be disappointed to learn that I was unsuccessful. I got close...a couple of fast feels in the front of his Cadillac.
—Bette Midler

Boys don't make passes at female smart-asses.
—Lettie Cottin Pogrebin

Early in my career I was in my dressing room making up. Suddenly, I turned around and there was this totally naked woman. "What's the matter, darling?" Tallulah Bankhead said. "Haven't you ever seen a blonde before?"
—Donald Sutherland

A woman will sometimes forgive the man who tries to seduce her, but never the man who misses an opportunity when offered.
—Talleyrand

It is not enough to conquer; one must know how to seduce.
—Voltaire

Come up and see me sometime.
> —Mae West

He who hesitates—is a damned fool.
> —Mae West

Sex Appeal

I'm not a homo and neither was John, but when I saw him come into a room, I got the jump you get when you see a beautiful girl. Being with him was electric, really electric.
> —Dan Aykroyd on John Belushi

Let's face it, when an attractive but aloof man comes along, there are some of us who offer to shine his shoes with our underpants.
> —Lynda Barry

Everybody's attracted to sex. So I'm learning to use it a lot better than I used to because if we ain't using it, we're wasting it.
> —Kim Basinger

One of the paramount reasons for staying attractive is so you can have somebody to go to bed with.
> —Helen Gurley Brown

Sweaty is sexy.
> —Farrah Fawcett

How he looks in a bathing suit should not be discounted. The fact is, I stare at men quite a lot.
> —Jane Fonda

Men ought to be more conscious of their bodies as an object of delight.

—Germaine Greer

I was probably the only revolutionary ever referred to as "cute."

—Abbie Hoffman

Sex appeal is 50 percent what you've got and 50 percent what people think you've got.

—Sophia Loren

You'd be surprised how much it costs to look this cheap.

—Dolly Parton

You'd be surprised how much better looking a man gets when you know he's worth a hundred and fifty million dollars.

—Joan Rivers

Women look forward to shopping for a bathing suit with the same anticipation that a baby seal looks forward to clubbing season.

—Rita Rudner

I enjoy that young girls in their twenties take an interest in me.

—Peter Sellers

She was all woman. She had curves in places other woman don't even have places.

—Cybill Shepherd on Marilyn Monroe

I know there are nights when I have the power, when I could put on something and walk in somewhere, and if there is a man who doesn't look at me, it's because he's gay.
—Kathleen Turner

I'm not a sexy person in real life.
—Tina Turner

It's better to be looked over than overlooked.
—Mae West

Sex Drive

His powers of recuperation are amazing. We made love all night long...we shared our fourth climax at dawn...and went frequently to 73rd Street where he fucked the daylights out of me....Was any woman ever happier?
—Lady Nancy Astor on George S. Kaufman

Most girls are reserved about getting down to it. They usually don't do it right away. But once they do it, women are bananas. They don't wanna do it, you can't make them do it, there's no way they'll do it—but once they do it, they won't let you alone.
—Mel Brooks

Male sexual response is far brisker and more automatic. It is triggered easily by things like putting a quarter in a vending machine.
—Alex Comfort

I started out to be a sex fiend, but I couldn't pass the physical.

—Robert Mitchum

Our biological drives are several million years older than our intelligence.

—Arthur E. Morgan

The sex drive is nothing but the motor memory of previously remembered pleasure.

—Wilhelm Reich

Marriage cannot cause happiness. Instead, it is always torture, which man has to pay for satisfying his sex urge.

—Leo Tolstoy

Sex Similes

Sex is like having dinner: sometimes you joke about the dishes, sometimes you take the meal seriously.

—Woody Allen

Sex is like money—very nice to have but vulgar to talk about.

—Tonia Berg

Sexual intercourse is kicking death in the ass while singing.

—Charles Bukowski

Conventional heterosexual intercourse is like squirting jam into a doughnut.

—Germaine Greer

Marrying a man is like buying something you've been admiring for a long time in a shop window. You may love it when you get it home, but it doesn't always go with everything else in the house.

—Jean Kerr

To say that you can love one person all your life is just like saying that one candle will continue burning as long as you live.

—Leo Tolstoy

Sailing is like screwing—you can never get enough.

—Ted Turner

Sex is like a small business; you gotta watch over it.

—Mae West

Sex Symbols

The most important sex symbol of all time.

—Brigitte Bardot on herself

Being a sex symbol is a heavy load, especially when one is tired, hurt, and bewildered.

—Clara Bow

Would it sound absurd if I said that in some sense I recoiled at the idea of being a sex symbol? I have broken hearts on both sides of the sexual equation.

—Dick Cavett

It's hard to figure how I got known as a sex symbol or brazen woman when I've been married most of my life.

—Cher

Three, four, five times a day every day was not unusual for [Warren Beatty], and he was also able to accept phone calls at the same time....Although it was exciting for the first few months, after a while, I found myself feeling somewhat like a sex object.

—Joan Collins

I wasn't erotic, I was snotty.

—Marlene Dietrich on why she
was a sex symbol

I think of myself as a sex symbol for men who don't give a damn.

—Phyllis Diller

A rampant cock. That's what I am to the world today, goddammit, a phallic symbol.

—Errol Flynn

It's rather amusing at my advanced age to become a sex symbol.

—John Forsythe

If I've still got my pants on in the second scene, I think they've sent me the wrong script.

—Mel Gibson

If I'm a release valve for women's pent-up feelings, that's great. It's as much a release for me as it is for them.

—Tom Jones

What's so fucking wrong with being a sex symbol?

—Kris Kristofferson

Once they call you a Latin lover, you're in real trouble. Women expect an Oscar performance in bed.
—Marcello Mastroianni

So what good is being a sex star if it drives your man away?
—Marilyn Monroe

A sex symbol becomes a thing. I hate being a thing.
—Marilyn Monroe

I've always wanted to be a sex symbol, but I don't think I am.... I can't imagine anyone thinking that I was sexually attractive. And if they do, where the fuck are they?
—Sinead O'Connor

Being a baldplate is an unfailing sex magnet.
—Telly Savalas

At first I loved it...in fact, I've always loved it. However, after you're pegged one, you learn—mainly through journalists—that maybe it's not such a good thing, that it has a shallow connotation.
—John Travolta

I love being a world-famous sex object. But I had to do a live show to show everybody I was more than just a cash register with glands.
—Raquel Welch

Being a sex symbol is rather like being a convict.
—Raquel Welch

Sexual Harassment

While you are away, movie stars are taking your women. Robert Redford is dating your girlfriend; Tom Selleck is kissing your lady; Bart Simpson is making love to your wife.

> —Baghdad Betty to Gulf War
> troops on Iraqi radio

There was physical abuse, there was emotional abuse, there was substance abuse.

> —Patti Davis on growing up
> with Nancy and Ronald
> Reagan

Woman is made the slave of a slave and is reckoned only fit for companionship in lust.

> —Eugene V. Debs

Many feminists would argue that as long as women are powerless relative to men, viewing "yes" as a sign of true consent is misguided.

> —Susan Estrich on why yes
> really means no

Thomas told me graphically of his own prowess....He spoke about acts he had seen in pornographic films.

> —Anita Hill on Clarence
> Thomas

The law recognizes that sexual harassment is a form of sex discrimination, which is certainly not confined to physical contact. Lewd looks and language are demeaning and degrading, and have long been used as a means of stereotyping women and girls and keeping them from experiencing the full range of opportunities available to men and boys in our society.

—Hubert H. Humphrey III

We're on this earth for one reason—to procreate, which means we are sexual objects.

—Joan Rivers

Sexual harassment on the job is not a problem for virtuous women.

—Phyllis Schlafly

In fact, he never did ask you to have sex, correct?

—Senator Alan Simpson to Anita Hill at the hearing for Supreme Court justice Clarence Thomas

They looked at you twice. Once to see your tits, and once to see what you can do.

—Carrie Snow on auditioning

Why are you wearing this? I can't see your breasts.

—Oliver Stone allegedly questioning a magazine reporter

Sexual Knowledge

Sex is identical to comedy in that it involves timing.

—Phyllis Diller

Johnny can't write about sex. He knows very little about it.

—Renee Grisham on her
bestselling author husband
John

If you want to read about love and marriage, you've got to buy two separate books.

—Alan King

I don't see much of Alfred any more since he got so interested in sex.

—Mrs. Alfred Kinsey

Males have made asses of themselves writing about the female sexual experience.

—William Masters

If sex is such a natural phenomenon, how come there are so many books on how to?

—Bette Midler

Children should never discuss sex in the presence of their elders.

—Gregory Nunn

When a girl can get birth control pills at age twelve, she knows as much as I do. My mom had stuff in her room that I could sneak in and get...books, vibrators. I did it. I'm sure everybody does.

—Prince

If the average parent knew as little about eating as he does about sex, he would quickly starve to death.

—Dr. David Reuben

I got all my information reading books; girls didn't talk to one another. Going down? I never knew what men were talking about.

—Joan Rivers

Defining bullshit as "nonsense" is bullshit.

—David Steinberg on the 1966
Random House Dictionary's
definition of "bullshit"

Sexual Preferences

Most middle-class and poor people envy the rich, never knowing the crosses we bear. We're alcoholics, high-class dope addicts, homosexuals and bisexuals. We fornicate strangely, we sleep with relatives.

—Alfred Bloomingdale

At certain times I like sex—like after a cigarette.

—Rodney Dangerfield

Personally, I like a woman to be a whore in bed.

—Bruce Dern

I'm a foreplay junkie.

—Richard Dreyfuss

Men want a woman whom they can turn on and off like a light switch.

—Ian Fleming

I prefer to be the mistress of a poor officer than a rich banker. It is my greatest pleasure to sleep with them without having to think of money....I like to make comparisons between various nationalities.
—Mata Hari

I like to wake up feeling a new man.
—Jean Harlow

I'm never through with a girl until I've had her three ways.
—John F. Kennedy

What man desires is a virgin who is a whore.
—Karl Kraus

Everyone probably thinks I'm a raving nymphomaniac, that I have an insatiable sexual appetite, when the truth is I'd rather read a book.
—Madonna

There are two things I like stiff, and one of them's Jell-O.
—Dame Nellie Melba

I always had a tremendous interest in big tits.
—Russ Meyer

Anyone who knows Dan Quayle knows he would rather play golf than have sex any day.
—Marilyn Quayle

Sex was best in the afternoon after a shower.
—Ronald Reagan

I am just an awkward old maid who has a very great attraction to men.

—Janet Reno on her sexual
preferences

Kissing, petting, and even intercourse are all right as long as they are sincere. I have never given a kiss in my life that wasn't sincere. As for intercourse, I'd say three times a day was about right.

—Margaret Sanger

I don't think a man is automatically great in bed if he goes on and on for ages. In fact, some of the most exciting times are when you just do it in five minutes.

—Cheryl Tiegs

I'd rather go to bed with Lillian Russell stark naked than Ulysses S. Grant in full military regalia.

—Mark Twain

All this fuss about sleeping together. For physical pleasure, I'd sooner go to my dentist any day.

—Evelyn Waugh

I like clean ladies and nice ladies.

—Lawrence Welk

Too much of a good thing is wonderful.

—Mae West

I like a man what takes his time.

—Mae West

According to the latest research, 60 percent of American couples are now screwing dog fashion—so both parties can watch television in bed.

—Billy Wilder

Sexually Transmitted Diseases

A knowledge of syphilis is not an instruction to contract it.

—Lenny Bruce

Uninhibited sex with multiple partners...is no longer possible because of the AIDS epidemic.

—Alex Comfort

The war against AIDS is the greatest public health emergency of our lifetime.

—Michael Dukakis

Despite a lifetime of service to the cause of sexual liberation, I have never caught venereal disease, which makes me feel rather like an Arctic explorer who has never had frostbite.

—Germaine Greer

You think if I had a sexual experience with another man, he wouldn't be a millionaire right now by coming out and saying that? We all know that he'd write a book, he'd be in the *Enquirer*, everything. He'd be a millionaire.

—Magic Johnson

In the age of AIDS, unprotected sex is reckless. But the truth is, I knew it then too. I just didn't pay attention.

—Magic Johnson

I used to carry penicillin tablets, because I have the greatest clap phobia of anyone in the world.

—Erica Jong

When they said, "Make love not war" at Woodstock, they never imagined that one would become as dangerous as the other.

—Jay Leno

I tried phone sex and it gave me an ear infection.

—Richard Lewis

Despite what we know about AIDS, you just think people will never die.

—Anthony Perkins

If I had to kiss a costar—because the disease is crossing over into the straight world—I'd want assurance he doesn't have AIDS. You have to protect yourself.

—Joan Rivers

Every man who has sexual relations with two women at the same time risks syphilis, even if the two women are faithful to him, for all libertine behavior spontaneously incites this disease.

—Alexander Weill (1891)

Toys

I'm through with men...I just want to be left alone with my vibrator. Yet another example of men being replaced by their machines.

—Lisa Alther

A plastic lady is no substitute. Plastic squeaks.
—Dudley Moore

There are a number of mechanical devices which increase sexual arousal, particularly in women. Chief among them is the Mercedes-Benz 380SL Convertible.
—P. J. O'Rourke

There, but for a typographical error, is the story of my life.
—Dorothy Parker when told that people were ducking for apples

I could take this home, Marilyn, this is something teenage boys might find of interest.
—Dan Quayle on a South American doll which displayed erecting male genitals

I'm romantic. I think every girl you go to bed with, you should be at least a little in love with. Otherwise, you might as well use a plastic dummy, or one of those jack-off machines.
—Burt Reynolds

Transsexuals

People who aren't sexually at peace with themselves tend to be uptight around me.
—Wendy/Walter Carlos

Being a women is of special interest only to aspiring male transsexuals. To actual women it is merely a good excuse not to play football.

—Fran Lebowitz

I didn't want to do away with the differences between the sexes. I am the living example of someone who wishes to maintain the polarity between the sexes.

—Transsexual Renée Richards

Virtue

Most plain girls are virtuous because of the scarcity of opportunity to be otherwise.

—Maya Angelou

It's the good girls who keep the diaries; the bad girls never have the time.

—Tallulah Bankhead

Rare are those who prefer virtue to the pleasures of sex.

—Confucius

A lady is one who never shows her underwear unintentionally.

—Lillian Day

Virtue is not photogenic.

—Kirk Douglas

A woman can look both moral and exciting...if she also looks as if it was quite a struggle.

—Edna Ferber

There's a fine line between being sweet and innocent and being a tough broad.
>—Phyllis George

I do not know if she was virtuous, but she was ugly, and with a woman that is half the battle.
>—Heinrich Heine

No matter which sex I went to bed with, I never smoked on the street.
>—Florence King

Morality is a disease which progresses in three ges: virtue—boredom—syphilis.
>—Karl Kraus

Puritanism...helps us enjoy our misery while we are inflicting it on others.
>—Marcel Ophuls

Whether a pretty woman grants or withholds her favors, she always likes to be asked for them.
>—Ovid

The modern rule is that every woman should be her own chaperon.
>—Amy Vanderbilt

It is one of the superstitions of the human mind to have imagined that virginity could be a virtue.
>—Voltaire

I wrote the story myself. It's about a girl who lost her reputation but never missed it.
>—Mae West

Goodness had nothing to do with it.

—Mae West on how she
obtained her diamonds

I'm never dirty. I'm interesting without being vulgar. I just...suggest.

—Mae West

Women with pasts interest men because they hope history will repeat itself.

—Mae West

I have bursts of being a lady, but it doesn't last long.

—Shelley Winters

Voyeurism

Naked children are so perfectly pure and lovely. I confess I do not admire boys. They always seem to me to need clothes; whereas one hardly sees why the lovely forms of girls should ever be covered up.

—Lewis Carroll

I see some of these magazines with naked guys standing around looking like real assholes and I wonder how any woman could get turned on.

—Cher

Women are like elephants to me—I like to look at them, but I wouldn't want to own one.

—W. C. Fields

Voyeurism is a healthy, nonparticipation sexual activity; the world should look at the world.

—Desmond Morris

Perhaps at fourteen every boy should be in love with some ideal woman to put on a pedestal and worship. As he grows up, of course, he will put her on a pedestal the better to view her legs.

—Barry Norman

I've nothing against sex, it's a marvelous human activity, but it was watching others do it all the time that got me down.

—John Trevelyan, British film
censor

Sex is more exciting on the screen than between the sheets.

—Andy Warhol

Women

Heav'n has no rage like love to hatred turned, nor hell a fury like a woman scorned.

—William Congreve

Being a woman is a terribly difficult trade, since it consists principally of dealing with men.

—Joseph Conrad

Nowadays you have the concept of the new woman. But the new woman is nothing without a man.

—Bob Dylan

The great question...which I have not been able to answer despite my thirty years in research into the feminine soul, is "What does a woman want?"
—Sigmund Freud

There are no bad women, some are better than others, but there are no bad ones.
—Buddy Hackett

Women are much less stable than men and much more promiscuous.
—Alfred Hitchcock

A woman is only a woman, but a good cigar is a smoke.
—Rudyard Kipling

Women complain about sex more often than men. Their gripes fall into two major categories; one, not enough; two, too much.
—Ann Landers

A woman is the only thing I am afraid of that I know will not hurt me.
—Abraham Lincoln

Strong women leave big hickeys.
—Madonna

I've always thought it's the role of women to spread sex and sunshine in the lives of men.
—Jayne Mansfield

Women, by nature, want to be dominated.
—Jayne Mansfield

I do not believe in using women in combat, because females are too fierce.

—Margaret Mead

If women didn't exist, all the money in the world would have no meaning.

—Aristotle Onassis

There are two kinds of women; those who want power in the world, and those who want power in bed.

—Jackie Kennedy Onassis

A woman is like a teabag. You can't tell how strong she is until you put her in hot water.

—Ronald Reagan

A woman without a man is like a fish without a bicycle.

—Gloria Steinem

I love women...my mother is a woman.

—Mike Tyson

Women are meant to be loved, not understood.

—Oscar Wilde

Women are a decorative sex; they never have anything to say, but they say it charmingly.

—Oscar Wilde

Women's Liberation

Real equality is going to come not when a female Einstein is recognized as quickly as a male Einstein, but when a female schlemiel is promoted as quickly as a male schlemiel.

—Bella Abzug

All men on my staff can type.

—Bella Abzug

It's babe power, which means you don't have to look, walk or act like a man to be his equal.

—Diane Brill on her book
*Boobs, Boys, and High
Heels—Or How to Get
Dressed in Just Under Six
Hours*

Nothing could induce me to vote for giving women the franchise. I am not going to be henpecked into a question of such importance.

—Winston Churchill

Sensible and responsible women do not want to vote.

—Grover Cleveland

Women are the only oppressed group in our society that live in intimate association with our oppressors.

—Evelyn Cunningham

A man's wife has more power over him than the state has.

—Ralph Waldo Emerson

185

The women's movement hasn't changed my life. It wouldn't dare.

—Zsa Zsa Gabor

Women who fancy they manipulate the world by pussy power and gentle cajolery are fools. It is slavery to have to adopt such tactics.

—Germaine Greer

During the feminist revolutions, the battle lines were again simple. It was easy to tell the enemy, he was the one with the penis. This is no longer strictly true. Some men are okay now. We're allowed to like them again. We still have to keep them in line, of course, but we no longer have to shoot them on sight.

—Cynthia Heimel

Beware of the man who praises women's liberation; he is about to quit his job.

—Erica Jong

I think if a woman has a right to an abortion and to control her body, then she has the right to exploit her body and make money from it. We have it hard enough. Why give up one of our major assets?

—Kathy Keeton

The people I'm furious with are the women's liberationists. They keep getting up on soapboxes and proclaiming women are brighter than men; that's true, but it should be kept quiet or it will ruin the whole racket.

—Anita Loos

Straight men need to be emasculated. I'm sorry. They need to be slapped around. Women have been kept down for too long. Every straight guy should have a man's tongue in his mouth at least once.

—Madonna

I want to be liberated and still be able to have a nice ass and shake it.

—Shirley MacLaine

Anyone who knows anything of history knows that great social changes are impossible without the feminine upheaval. Social progress can be measured exactly by the social position of the fair sex; the ugly ones included.

—Karl Marx

The women's liberation warriors think they have something new, but it's just their armies coming out of the hills. Sweet women ambushed men always, at their cradles, in the kitchen, in the bedroom.

—Mario Puzo

Scratch most feminists and underneath there is a woman who longs to be a sex object; the difference is that it is not all she longs to be.

—Betty Rollins

No one should ever have to dance backwards all their lives.

—Jill Ruckelshaus

I'm all for the ERA. I want to see women equal to men— not so damn superior like they have been.

—Nipsey Russell

I believe woman is enslaved...by sex conventions, by motherhood and its present necessary childbearing, by wage-slavery, by middle-class morality.
—Margaret Sanger

The claim that American women are downtrodden and unfairly treated is the fraud of the century.
—Phyllis Schlafly

Women's degradation is man's idea of his sexual rights. Our religion, laws, customs, are all founded on the belief that woman was made for man.
—Elizabeth Cady Stanton

Will there be sex after liberation?
—Gloria Steinem

I have yet to hear a man ask for advice on how to combine marriage and a career.
—Gloria Steinem

The only trouble with sexually liberating women is that there aren't enough sexually liberated men to go around.
—Gloria Steinem

A woman reading *Playboy* feels a little like a Jew reading a Nazi manual.
—Gloria Steinem

I can't mate in captivity.
—Gloria Steinem

A liberated woman is one who has sex before marriage and a job after.
—Gloria Steinem

I owe nothing to women's lib.

>—Margaret Thatcher

Men are irrelevant. Women are happy or unhappy, fulfilled or unfulfilled, and it has nothing to do with men.

>—Fay Weldon

The women's movement....would probably move more quickly if men were running it.

>—Jimmy Williams

Index

Index

Carter, Billy, *brother of Jimmy Carter,* 47

Carter, Jimmy, *U.S. president,* 76, 161

Carter, Lillian, *mother of Jimmy Carter,* 32

Casanova, *Italian adventurer and seductor,* 1, 49

Cassidy, Butch, *outlaw,* 59

Cavett, Dick, *TV talk-show host,* 37, 167

Chamberlain, Lord, *British politician and statesman,* 63

Chamberlain, Wilt, *basketball player,* 149

Chambers, Marilyn, *porn actress,* 53, 81, 82

Chaplin, Charlie, *silent-film star,* 93, 153, 161

Charles, Prince, *British royal,* 53, 71, 144

Chaucer, Geoffrey, *poet,* 32

Cher, *singer, actress,* 7, 37, 61, 89, 97, 124, 149, 167, 181

Chesterfield, Fourth Earl of, *British statesman and writer,* 113

Chevalier, Maurice, *actor,* 37, 89

Child, Julia, *chef,* 61

Children's Sex Manual, 128

Chopin, Frederic, *composer,* 38

Chrisholm, Shirley, *congresswoman,* 19

Christie, Agatha, *mystery writer,* 7

Churchill, Winston, *politician and statesman,* 185

Clancy, Tom, *writer,* 63, 97

Cleaver, Eldridge, *black activist,* 63

Cleveland, Grover, *U.S. president,* 185

Clinton, Bill, *U.S. president,* 47, 120

Clinton, Hillary Rodham, *first lady,* 146

Coleridge, Samuel Taylor, *English poet and philosopher,* 97

Collins, Jackie, *novelist,* 19

Collins, Joan, *actress,* 168

Collins, Nancy, *journalist,* 82

Colson, Charles, *presidential aide,* 41

Comfort, Alex, *sexologist, writer,* 1, 14, 32, 114, 165, 176

Confucious, *Chinese philosopher,* 179

Congreve, William, *British playwright,* 182

Connors, Jimmy, *tennis player,* 114

Conrad, Joseph, *writer,* 19, 182

Coolidge, Calvin, *U.S. president,* 136

Cooper, Alice, *rock singer,* 51, 54

Cooper, Jackie, *actor,* 55

Copeland, Harlon, *county sheriff,* 42

Corelli, Marie, *British novelist,* 97

Cort, David, *writer,* 153

Costa, Dr. Paul T., *psychologist,* 14

Coward, Noel, *British playwright,* 139

Crahan, Dr. Marcus, *physician,* 26

Crawford, Joan, *actress,* 59, 89, 146

Cresson, Edith, *French politician,* 23, 69

Crisp, Quentin, *British writer,* 132

Cunningham, Evelyn, *feminist,* 185

Curtis, Jamie Lee, *actress,* 23, 120

Curtis, Tony, *actor,* 86

Cutter, Devorah, *writer, director,* 93

Dahlberg, Edward, *writer,* 94

Daltry, Roger, *British rock singer,* 50

Dangerfield, Rodney, *comedian,* 7, 54, 76, 82, 98, 126, 132, 173

Darrow, Clarence, *lawyer,* 26, 51

Daulton, Darren, *baseball player,* 17

da Vinci, Leonardo, *artist and scientist,* 14, 15, 133

Davis, Bette, *actress,* 34, 55, 59, 73, 98, 114

Davis, Elizabeth Gould, *writer,* 15

Davis, Patti, *writer,* 170

Day, Doris, *actress,* 17, 36, 144

Day, Lillian, *writer,* 179

Dean, James, *actor,* 69

Debs, Eugene V., *labor organizer,* 170

DeConcini, Dennis, *U.S. senator,* 136

Delano, Lynn, *prison official,* 142

Democritus, *Greek philosopher,* 128

Deneuve, Catherine, *actress,* 23

Denton, Jeremiah, *U.S. senator,* 156

Dern, Bruce, *actor,* 173

Detremerie, Jean Pierre, *Belgian politician,* 76

Diana, Princess, *British royal,* 17

Dickinson, Angie, *actress,* 34

Dietrich, Marlene, *actress,* 2, 9, 10, 19, 105, 114, 168

Diller, Phyllis, *comedian,* 2, 10, 23, 38, 76, 168, 171

Diplock, Lord, *British lawyer,* 30

Disney, Walt, *cartoonist, amusement park tycoon,* 89

Disraeli, Benjamin, *British politician and statesman,* 98, 107

Douglas, Kirk, *actor,* 147, 179

Downey, Robert, Jr., *British professor of moral philosophy,* 159

Dreyfus, Richard, *actor,* 173

Drury, Ian, *British rock musician,* 133

duc d'Aumale, Henri, *French soldier,* 7

Dukakis, Michael, *governor,* 176

Duke of Windsor, *British royal,* 9

Dumas, Alexandre, *French playwright,* 2, 19, 77, 89

Duncan, Isadora, *dancer,* 98

Dunn, Dr. Charles Hunter, *medical doctor, Harvard U.,* 104

Durst, Will, *comedian,* 159

Dylan, Bob, *singer, songwriter,* 182

Easton, Sheena, *singer,* 162

Eastwood, Clint, *actor,* 19

Edwards, Edwin C., *governor of Louisiana,* 136

Einstein, Albert, *physicist,* 158

Ekland, Britt, *actress,* 77, 114, 128

Elizabeth, Queen, I, *British Royal,* 32

Ellington, Duke, *musician,* 89

Ellis, Dr. Albert, *psychologist,* 77

Emerson, Ralph Waldo, *essayist, poet, philosopher,* 114, 185

Ephron, Nora, *writer,* 105

Estrich, Susan, *feminist,* 170

Exodus 20, 2

Fairchild, Morgan, *actress,* 131

Faldo, Nick, *British golfer,* 98

Faulkner, William, *writer,* 144

Fawcett, Farrah, *actress,* 19, 163

Feiffer, Jules, *cartoonist,* 71

Feinstein, Bruce, *writer,* 128

Ferber, Edna, *writer,* 179

Ferris, Richard J., *business executive,* 142

Index

Felner, P. Jay, *student*, 156

Fields, W. C., *juggler, actor*, 2, 44, 47, 61, 114, 119, 120, 181

Fisher, Eddie, *singer*, 162

Fitzgerald, F. Scott, *writer*, 86

Fleming, Ian, *writer*, 7, 94, 173

Flowers, Gennifer, *alleged adulteress with Bill Clinton*, 59, 77, 120

Flynn, Errol, *actor*, 168

Flynt, Larry, *porn magazine publisher*, 30, 159

Fonda, Jane, *actress*, 54, 107, 163

Ford, Betty, *first lady*, 144

Forsythe, John, *actor*, 168

Foxe, Fanne, *stripper*, 49

Foxx, Red, *comedian, actor*, 155

Francis, Brenden, *writer*, 153

Franklin, Benjamin, *statesman, scientist*, 2, 988

French proverb, 162

French, Marilyn, *novelist*, 156

Freud, Sigmond, *Austrian psychoanalyst*, 13, 63, 89, 105, 133, 183

Friedman, Bruce Jay, *writer*, 49, 128

Frisch, Max, *Swiss novelist and playwright*, 82

Fromm, Erich, *psychologist*, 90

Gable, Clark, *actor*, 90, 149

Gabor, Zsa Zsa, *actress*, 45, 46, 65, 73, 77, 81, 98, 99, 105, 106, 186

Galbraith, John Kenneth, *economist*, 115

Gardner, Ava, *actress*, 86

Gardner, John Nance, *U.S. vice president*, 136

Garrett, Johnny Frank, *convicted murderer*, 42

Gass, William, *writer*, 139

Geldof, Bob, *music-business entrepreneur*, 109

George, Boy, *British rock singer*, 28, 38, 69, 124

George, Phyllis, *TV commentator*, 180

Getty, J. Paul, *oil tycoon*, 80

Gibson, Mel, *actor*, 168

Gifford, Kathy Lee, *singer, talk-show host*, 160

Gilder, George, *writer*, 49

Gilman, Charlotte Perkins, *writer*, 10

Gingold, Hermione, *British actress*, 34

Ginsberg, Allen, *poet*, 50

Glaven, Ed, *TV producer*, 153

Glyn, Anthony, *British writer*, 129

Goldstein, Al, *editor, porn reviewer*, 77, 139, 147, 159

Goldwater, Barry, *U.S. senator*, 17, 67, 120, 136, 150

Goldwyn, Sam, *movie producer*, 17, 115

Goodell, Charles, *U.S. senator*, 136

Goodman, Paul, *writer*, 133

Gordon, Sol, *writer*, 140

Gore, Tipper, *wife of Al Gore*, 75

Grable, Betty, *actress*, 10

Grace, Peter, *businessman*, 120

Graham, Billy, *evangelist*, 10, 156

Grant, Cary, *actor*, 61

Grant, Lee, *actress*, 38

Grant, Ulysses S., *U.S. president*, 109

Greenburg, Dan, *writer*, 90

Greer, Germaine, *writer, feminist*, 11, 24, 54, 74, 90, 94, 106, 164, 166, 176, 186

Griffiths, Trevor, *British playwright*, 58

Grisham, Renee, *wife of John Grisham*, 172

Grizzard, Lewis, *journalist, writer*, 46, 51

Guccione, Bob, *porn-magazine publisher*, 56

Gwynn, Nell, *actress*, 159

Hackett, Buddy, *comedian*, 104, 183

Haig, Alexander, *U.S. army general, presidential aide*, 42

Haitt, Gail, *hairdresser*, 24

Hall, Arsenio, *TV talk-show host*, 83

Hall, Jerry, *model*, 2, 77, 81, 124

Hamilton, George, *actor*, 111

Hamm, Stephen, *Dutch scientist*, 129

Harding, Tonya, *figure skater*, 38

Harding, Warren G., *U.S. president*, 150

Hari, Mata, *spy*, 174

Harlow, Bryce N., *presidential aide*, 17

Harlow, Jean, *actress*, 94, 174

Hart, Gary, *U.S. senator*, 72

Haskell, Molly, *writer*, 150

Hatch, Orrin, *U.S. senator*, 63

Hawkins, Jay, *British rock star*, 15

Hawn, Goldie, *actress*, 83, 150

Hawthorne, Nathanial, *writer*, 32

Head, Edith, *manners expert*, 34

Heatherton, Joey, *actress*, 133

Hefner, Hugh, *porn-magazine publisher*, 9, 28, 38, 99, 140, 159

Heimel, Cynthia, *writer*, 35, 159, 186

Heine, Heinrich, *German poet, writer*, 99, 109, 180

Heller, Joseph, *writer*, 46, 49

Hellman, Lillian, *playwright*, 15

Hemingway, Ernest, *writer*, 72, 86, 129

Hepburn, Katharine, *actress*, 24, 36, 38

Hesburgh, Theodore, *university president*, 155

Hill, Anita, *law professor*, 170

Hillingdon, Lady Alice, *British noblewoman*, 74

Hinckley, John, *would-be assassin*, 42

Hipponax, *Greek philosopher*, 44

Hitchcock, Alfred, *movie producer, director*, 7, 83, 183

Hitler, Adolph, *German chancellor*, 73

Hoffa, Jimmy, *labor leader*, 121

Hoffman, Abbie, *political activist*, 164

Holiday, Billie, *blues singer*, 51

Hollander, Xaviera, *sex-advice columnist*, 15, 38, 50, 54, 61, 62, 78, 126, 129, 155

Holmes, John, *porn actor*, 104

Holmes, Oliver Wendell, *Supreme Court justice*, 20

Hoover, J. Edgar, *FBI director*, 126, 145

Hope, Bob, *comedian, actor*, 17, 86, 159

Hornung, Paul, *football player*, 2, 147

Howe, Gordie, *hockey player*, 146

Hudson, Rock, *actor*, 28, 50, 64

Hughes, Howard, *industrialist, movie producer*, 11

Hugo, Victor, *French writer*, 2

Humperdinck, Engelbert, *singer*, 142

Humphrey, Hubert H., III, *politician*, 171

Huneker, James G., *musician, critic*, 32

Hutton, Lauren, *model, actress*, 99, 147

Huxley, Aldous, *British writer*, 33

Idle, Eric, *British comedian, actor*, 3

Index